Racquetball Today

Racquetball Today

Second Edition

Lynn Adams

Women's Professional Racquetball Champion
Libertyville, Illinois

Erwin Goldbloom

Retired Chairperson, Physical Education Department
Los Angeles Pierce College

Series Editor
Bob O'Connor, Ed. D.

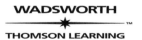

WADSWORTH

™

THOMSON LEARNING

Australia • Canada • Mexico • Singapore • Spain • United Kingdom • United States

WADSWORTH

THOMSON LEARNING ™

Publisher: Peter Marshall
Associate Editor: April Lemons
Marketing Manager: Joanne Terhaar
Assistant Editor: John Boyd
Editorial Assistant: Andrea Kesterke
Project Editor: Sandra Craig
Print Buyer: April Reynolds
Permissions Editor: Stephanie Keough-Hedges

Production and Composition: Carlisle Communications
Interior and Cover Design: Harry Voigt Graphic Design
Copy Editor: Mark Spann
Printer: Webcom

Wadsworth/Thomson Learning
10 Davis Drive
Belmont, CA 94002-3098
USA

For more information about our products, contact us:

Thomson Learning Academic Resource Center
1-800-423-0563
http://www.wadsworth.com

International Headquarters
Thomson Learning
International Division
290 Harbor Drive, 2nd Floor
Stamford, CT 06902-7477
USA

UK/Europe/Middle East/South Africa
Thomson Learning
Berkshire House
168-173 High Holborn
London WC1V 7AA
United Kingdom

Asia
Thomson Learning
60 Albert Street #15-01
Albert Complex
Singapore 189969

Canada
Nelson Thomson Learning
1120 Birchmount Road
Toronto, Ontario M1K 5G4
Canada

Library of Congress Cataloging-in-Publication Data

Adams, Lynn.
    Racquetball today / Lynn Adams, Erwin Goldbloom.—
    2nd ed. p. cm.
    Includes index.
    ISBN 0-534-55234-X
    1. Racquetball.   I. Goldbloom, Erwin.   II. Title.

GV1003.34 .A29 2001
796.343—dc21   00-049531

Contents

Preface

This text is intended to assist players—beginning, intermediate and advanced—who are interested in becoming complete racquetball players. While most people can play racquetball after a few instructional sessions, to be able to play well, a person should become a student of the game, continually learning and improving in all areas.

Racquetball Today provides the necessary learning tools for the beginning player. The text then progresses to build strategies and drills for the intermediate and advanced players. The varied aspects of the game—necessary shots, correct footwork, body positioning, winning strategies, mental preparedness and physical conditioning—are all discussed. Skills are explained completely and are reinforced by a series of photographs and illustrations that isolate the various parts of each shot. The chapters contain checklists to help the player retain vital information. Now, all the player has to add is practice.

The correct technique is the most important element in playing consistent racquetball. While there may be different opinions regarding the execution of certain skills, the authors have attempted to present methods developed by the top players in the world. The explanation of methods is fully supported by the illustration program for the text.

Emphasis in *Racquetball Today* has been placed on providing the player with the versatility to become a complete racquetball player. Comprehensive chapters cover all the important aspects of the game, which include service returns, backwall play, mental approach, the three-wall game, and drills. Also included are chapters on physical fitness and weight training, providing instruction specific to the sport.

Acknowledgments

The development of this text could not have progressed without the helpful criticisms and suggestions from colleagues reviewing the manuscript. The authors gratefully acknowledge:

Peter P. Bolen, Colorado State University
Mike Bobo, Texas Tech University
Lynn Cherry, California State University, Sacramento
Don Hester, University of Florida
Noel Maldonado, California State University, Los Angeles
Toby McCammon, Johnson County Community College
Jay Moxley, California State University, Los Angeles

Angela N. Smith, University of Arkansas, Fayetteville
Norris Stevenson, St. Louis Community College
Todd D. Williams, University of Puget Sound
Elaine Budde, Roanoke College

The authors also are grateful to Jim Carson for all his help and racquetball knowledge and to John Muir for his contributions to the chapter on the three-wall game.

Additionally, the authors would like to thank the players who served as models for the text photographs and David Hanover for his excellent photography.

Now, learn—play—and enjoy the game of racquetball!

Introduction to the Game

Racquetball is an exciting game that gives players an opportunity to have fun from the very first day. It becomes more and more enjoyable as the player's skill increases through the intermediate level into the advanced and tournament levels.

A good racquetball session will provide a person with an effective cardiovascular workout, which is healthy for the body. The competitive nature of the game, the physical demands, and the hitting action also make racquetball a stress reducer, adding extensive mental, social, and emotional benefits as well.

Step on a court and with a few minutes of basic instruction, one can be ready to play. The basic playing rules are simple: players alternate hitting the ball to the front wall before it hits the floor a second time, and only the server can score. Easy enough?

The game can be played indoors (four-wall) or outdoors (usually three-wall), by people of any age, even the physically handicapped. It is certainly a game for all seasons.

History

Racquetball evolved from handball, a four-wall, indoor court game, and other racquet games such as tennis and badminton. There are some similarities with squash, which is also played in an enclosed court with racquets. However, the national popularity of racquetball has far outdistanced these earlier counterparts.

Court games have been with us for many centuries. They were common in various cultures throughout the world. Racquets were introduced a few centuries ago, when tennis began to make inroads among the French aristocracy.

The game of handball was brought to the United States from Ireland in the nineteenth century, an adaptation of an earlier British game called fives. It evolved into a game called paddleball, which was played with wooden paddles on handball courts. In the 1940s, the paddles gave way to short racquets strung like tennis racquets, called paddle-rackets.

It was not until 1969, in St. Louis, Missouri, that the name of the game was changed to *racquetball* and the International Racquetball Association was formed. At that time Robert Kendler, the founder and former president of the United States Handball Association, became the president of the International Racquetball Association (IRA).

Since racquetball rules required the use of handball courts, a conflict arose over who had priority for their use. The YMCA, private handball clubs, and some schools banned racquetball players from their handball facilities. This necessitated the development of new facilities, usually private, for the rapidly growing number of racquetball players.

In 1973, Kendler resigned his post with IRA and started the National Racquetball Club (NRC). This group sponsored the first professional racquetball tour, as well as the United States Racquetball Association (USRA) for amateur players. In late 1979, professional women players formed the Women's Professional Racquetball Association (WPRA) to promote the progress of women in the sport. The WPRA held the first women-only event in January 1980, in Rockville, New York. The men's and women's tours have been separate entities from that time.

Racquetball has made an impact on society, providing a new avenue for individuals to participate in a rewarding activity and to improve physical conditioning. It also is having an effect upon the marketplace.

Equipment

The shape of equipment changed rapidly from the first crude racquets. The material has become lighter, stronger, and more colorful, and the stringing has become tighter to provide added power. The balls have become livelier and the clothes flashier. Racquetball has arrived on the fitness scene and is making a dent in the multi-million dollar sportswear and fitness club industries.

Summary

1. Racquetball gives players an opportunity to have fun from the first day.
2. The game went through many changes while evolving into its modern look.
3. The game has financially affected society by shaping health clubs, advancing the technology of game-related equipment, and updating the design of game-related sportswear.

1   *Equipment*

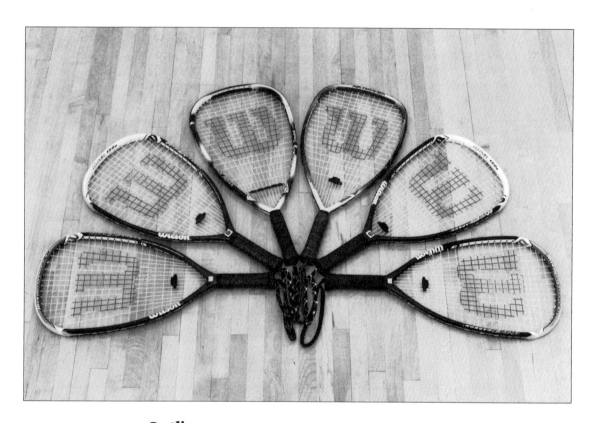

Outline

The good news is that the cost of racquetball gear is relatively low when compared with other recreational sports gear. All one really needs to play is a racquet, a ball, protective eyewear, shorts, a T-shirt, socks, and a pair of tennis or other court shoes. No special uniform or dress is required. All the equipment needed can fit into a small athletic bag.

After playing the game for a while, many people are bitten by the "racquetball bug" and want to purchase equipment specifically designed for each individual's type of game or personality.

Selecting a Racquet

The first concern of the player is obtaining a racquet. Racquets can range in price from $10 to $250, but it is not necessary to purchase an expensive model when beginning to learn the game. Wait until you develop a definite style of play before deciding what type of racquet will best suit your game.

Manufacturers have matched the increased popularity of racquetball (and the fitness craze in general) with space-age technology. The trend in racquets has moved away from the early wood-frame racquets (now obsolete and banned on many courts), to lighter-weight aluminum, fiberglass, and graphite and boron composites.

Generally speaking, aluminum and fiberglass racquets are more flexible and emphasize control, while composite racquets, which are lighter than aluminum and fiberglass, are stiffer and more power-oriented.

Racquets may not be over 22 inches in length and must have a thong, which attaches to the player's wrist. This thong, when slipped over the wrist, prevents the racquet from accidentally slipping and injuring another player. If someone tries to play without wearing the thong, it is the prerogative of the other player *not* to play.

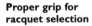

Proper grip for racquet selection

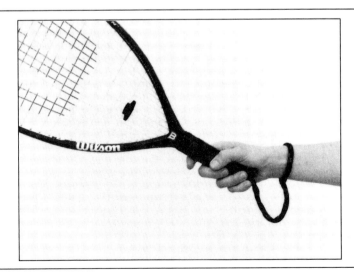

Racquet shapes and styles

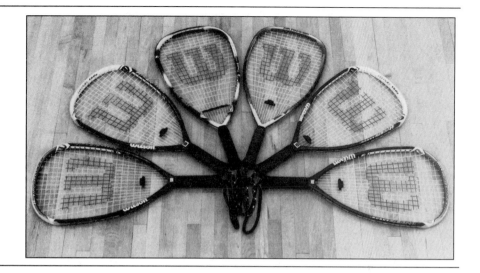

Realizing individual preferences, racquets are made in different sizes, degrees of flexibility, head shapes and sizes, string patterns, colors, and grip sizes. When selecting a racquet, one of the most important factors is grip size. A smaller circumference will enable one to attain the flexible wrist action necessary to become a complete player. To check for proper fit, simply hold the racquet, allowing the middle and ring fingers to lightly contact the fleshy part of your lower thumb (see photo on page 2). Most racquets have the grip size embossed on the base of the handle. Grips are constructed primarily of leather or rubber. Each kind of grip has its advocates among players.

The important thing is to choose a racquet that fits your individual style of play. Take time to select a racquet that feels comfortable when held in your hand and while swinging. There is an advantage to trying a certain type of racquet on the court. Many clubs provide "demo" racquets to help you make a choice.

Hard-hitters usually select a stiffer racquet, while a control-oriented player will choose a more flexible one for that special touch.

Racquets are designed with two basic head shapes: teardrop and quadriform. The teardrop style generally produces stiffer frames and places the sweet spot farther from the handle, where the added leverage generates more power, while the quadriform head shape centers the sweet spot, enabling the player to have more control for shot placement.

String Tension

The *strings* are usually 15 gauge nylon, and the tension will vary to match each type of racquet and style. Oversized racquets are strung with more tension than mid-sized racquets, and the modern composite racquets are strung with more tension than the older ones. Each racquet is designed for a specific string tension, which is designated by the manufacturer.

Protective Eyewear

The use of eyeguards or protective glasses is strongly recommended by the authors. In fact, professionals won't even get on the court without them, and believe that their wear should be mandatory. When playing in a sanctioned United States Racquetball Association (USRA) tournament, protective, lensed eyewear *is* mandatory. While protecting a player's most precious assets, the eyes, protective eyewear allows the player to follow the flight of the ball around the court throughout the rally without being hit in the eye by an errant shot.

There are two types of eyewear. One type is plastic with open slots, rather than lenses, to see through. These goggles have no distortion, but do not provide as much protection as lensed eyewear because the ball can fit through one of the openings when it becomes compressed on impact. Lensed eyewear have unbreakable shatterproof lenses and are mandatory for USRA tournament play. If corrective vision is needed, prescription safety glasses can be made or contact lenses may be worn beneath standard safety goggles.

Other Equipment

Gloves are worn by most players to reduce the possibility of the racquet slipping in the hand due to perspiration. These lightweight gloves, similar to baseball batting gloves or golfing gloves, are made of sheepskin, synthetic leather, or calfskin. Serious players who play for long periods usually have several gloves so as to change as each glove gets wet.

Proper eyewear
Three types shown: plastic eyewear with open slots, goggles, pair of lensed glasses

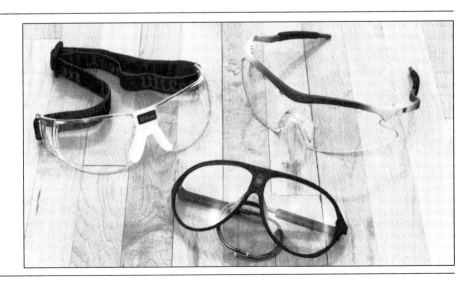

Other equipment

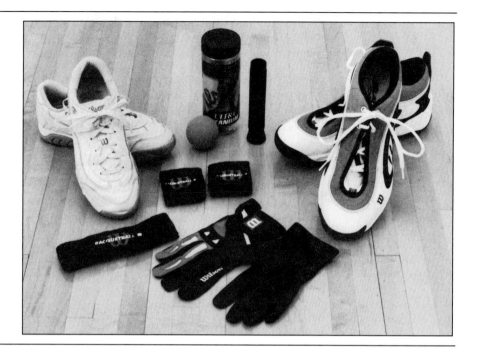

Sweat bands on the wrist are popular with racquetball players to keep water from wetting the hand or glove and on the forehead to stop the perspiration from getting into the eyes.

Shoes

While any kind of tennis shoe is adequate to play racquetball, a pair of sturdy, well-fitting shoes with good support are recommended. Shoe manufacturers have developed shoes designed specifically for the demands of racquetball play. Avoid aching, blistered feet and twisted ankles by selecting shoes that will give both comfort and support. Black-soled shoes are banned at all indoor facilities because they mark the floor, and running shoes are not recommended due to the lack of lateral support, a possible cause of injury to ankles.

Balls

The ball used in racquetball must be 2 1/4 inches in diameter, weigh approximately 1.4 ounces, and bounce 68 to 70 inches from a 100-inch drop. Manufacturers guarantee consistency, and the balls are easily obtained at many retail outlets for about one dollar a ball.

The original ball, (called a "Pinky,") which was made from the core of a tennis ball, proved to be too lively and was soon replaced by a black, less bouncy ball. The current color, blue, is used to make it easier to see the ball. Almost as

Checklist for Equipment Selection

1. Select a racquet to fit your individual style of play.
2. Grip size is an important factor in racquet selection.
3. Grip size may be checked by making sure that the middle and ring fingers lightly contact the fleshy part of the thumb.
4. Select USRA recommended protective eyewear.
5. Select comfortable shoes that allow for lateral support.
6. Other equipment needed are a glove, a ball, loose comfortable clothing, and a bag to hold the equipment.

popular as the blue ball, is the green ball. It is used exclusively on the men and women's pro tour events.

For a relatively small initial cash outlay, one can be introduced to the game of racquetball. A racquet, ball, glove, protective eyewear, and normal athletic clothing are all that are required.

Summary

1. Racquetball equipment is relatively inexpensive.
2. Racquets have followed the high-tech trend from wooden, aluminum, and fiberglass racquets to graphite-boron composites that are designed to meet individual differences in playing styles.
3. Protective eyewear helps to make racquetball a safer sport, by protecting a player's eyes from the most dangerous racquetball-related injury.
4. There is relatively little equipment needed to get involved in the sport: a racquet, balls, eyewear, a glove, loose-fitting athletic clothes, and sturdy, comfortable athletic shoes, which allow lateral movement.

2 *Let's Play*

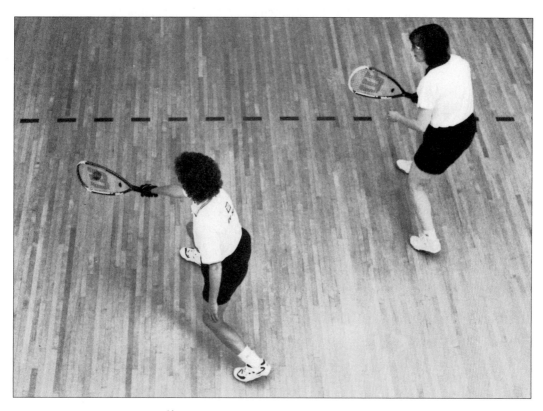

Outline

N ow that we have the equipment together, it's time to get out on the court and begin to play. But first, let's take a quick look at how to play the game.

The Rules

The game is played on an enclosed court that is 40 feet long, 20 feet wide, and 20 feet high. After the service, the ball can hit any surface, including the back wall and ceiling, as long as it eventually hits the front wall before the ball hits the floor a second time.

The Singles Game

The basic rule of racquetball is that players alternate hitting the ball to the front wall before it hits the floor a second time, and only the server scores. To begin play, one player (the *server*) puts the ball in play, and the other player (the *receiver*) waits to begin the rally. The game is over when either player reaches fifteen points, or eleven points if in a tie-breaker.

The Service

Play begins with the serving player standing anywhere within the service zone—a 5 × 20 foot area. Both of the server's feet must remain in the service zone until the ball passes the *short line,* which is the rear line of the service zone. After the server calls the score, always giving the server's score first (e.g., if the server has 6 points and the opponent has 8, the call is "6–8"), the ball is dropped to the floor and must be hit on the first bounce directly to the front wall. The server has ten seconds from the time the score is called to deliver the serve.

In order to be a valid serve, the ball must always hit the front wall first and on the rebound touch the floor behind the short line (either with or without touching one side wall). After this sequence, the serve can touch another wall and/or the back wall. If the ball hits the floor a second time before being returned to the front wall, it is a point; an *ace* for the server.

Illegal Serves

If a served ball hits the floor, a side wall, or the ceiling before hitting the front wall, it results in an immediate loss of service—an *out serve.* A serve that hits the server is also an out serve.

The following serves are fault serves: short, long, three-wall, ceiling, foot fault, and screen serves. Two consecutive fault serves result in loss of service.

A served ball that hits the front wall but also hits the floor before passing the short line is a *short serve.* (By the way, serves that land on the line are also

Diagram for indoor court with measurements

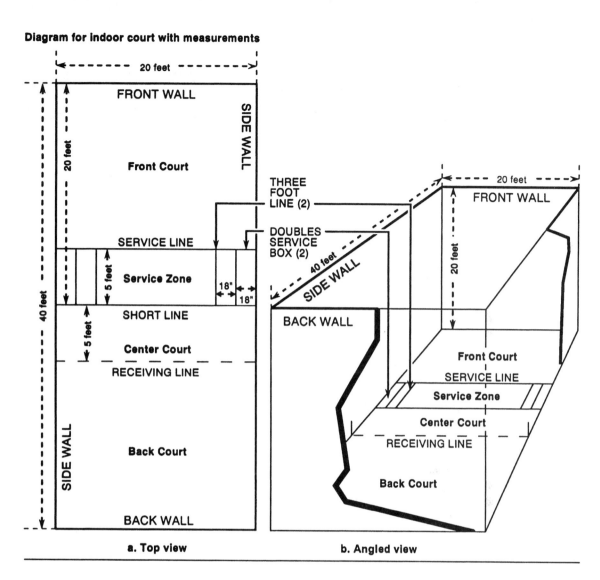

a. Top view

b. Angled view

Starting position for singles

Server (1) may stand anywhere in service zone

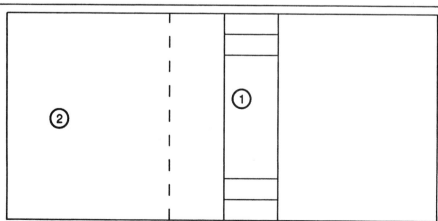

1 = server   2 = receiver

Checklist for Illegal Serves

Illegal Serves

1. Dead ball serves (Serve again; no penalty)
   - Fault (open—one more attempt)
   - Court hinders
   - Broken ball

2. Fault serves (two consecutive fault serves result in side out or hand out)
   Except open—one serve
   - Foot faults
   - Short serve
   - Three-wall serve
   - Ceiling serve
   - Long serve
   - Bouncing ball outside serve
   - Out serve
   - Illegal drive serve
   - Screen serve
   - Serving before the receiver is ready
   - Partner not in doubles box (Doubles)
   - Served ball hits partner not in doubles box (Doubles)

3. Out serves (results in an out; loss of service)
   - Two consecutive fault serves (one serve in open)
   - Missed serve attempt
   - Touched serve (ball touches server on fly)
   - Fake or balk serves
   - Illegal hit (ball hit twice or with handle or body)
   - Non-front wall serves (ball hits floor, side wall or ceiling before front wall)
   - Crotch serve (ball hits in side wall corner)
   - Out of court serve
   - Safety zone violation (doubles)
   - Out-of-order serve (doubles)
   - Ball hits partner outside of doubles box

considered short.) A served ball that hits the rear wall before touching the floor is a *long serve.* If it hits any two side walls before the floor, it is a *three-wall serve,* or if it hits the ceiling after contacting the front wall, it is a *ceiling serve.*

When the server steps out of the service zone before the ball has passed the short line, it is considered a *foot fault.* If the serve is legal but passes so close to the server as to obstruct the view of the receiver, it is a screen serve. A three-foot line violation is a type of *screen serve;* this rule prohibits a player from hitting a drive serve (a low, hard serve) inside of that three-foot zone.

Checklist for Legal Serves

Legal Serve
1. Server must hit ball after only one bounce
2. Server may not hit ball on the fly (before it bounces)
3. Server must remain within the serving zone until ball passes the short line
4. Ball must be served within 10 seconds
5. Ball must hit front wall directly from the racquet
6. Ball may hit the front wall and then one side wall before bouncing on the floor
7. Ball must rebound from the front wall and land in the area behind the short line before hitting the back wall or a second side wall

Legal Serves

To be a legal serve, the ball must hit the front wall directly from the serve and land in the twenty-foot square area toward the rear of the court before hitting more than one side wall or the back wall. Hitting the ceiling is not considered a legal serve.

Now the receiver of a legal serve must return the ball to the front wall before it again touches the floor. Any combination of walls and ceiling, in any order, may be used as long as the ball contacts the front wall before again touching the floor.

Return of Serve

The *receiving line* is a line five feet behind the short line, often marked by a small vertical line on the side wall or by a broken line on the floor. The receiver may not hit the serve until the ball has passed, bounced, or crossed this line, or the server will win the point. Neither the receiver nor the racquet may break the plane of the receiving line when making contact with the ball, but once contact has been made, the follow-through can enter the zone. Although the receiver must wait until the serve has passed the receiving line before hitting the ball, there is the option of hitting it before or after the first bounce. (For the complete United States Racquetball Association rules, see Appendix A.)

Scoring

Now the rally is on and both players have the same opportunities to utilize the entire court. As mentioned before, only the server can score. The game is over when one of the players reaches *15 points.* Unlike some other games, in

Checklist for Scoring

1. The server scores a point if the receiver's return shot fails to hit the front wall before it hits the floor.
2. Once a rally has begun, the server scores a point whenever the receiver fails to return the ball to the front wall after the ball has been hit by the server.
3. *Only* the server may score a point.
4. The receiver becomes the server if the server fails to make a legal serve, or if during a rally the server fails to return the receiver's shot to the front wall before it hits the floor.
5. The game is ended when a player reaches 15 points.
6. In tournament play, when both players win one game, the third game is called a tie-breaker and is played until either player reaches 11 points.

racquetball the player who reaches the game score first is the winner. The winner does not have to win by two points; 14–14 is game point for both players.

In tournament play, when both players or teams win one game, a tie-breaker is played to 11 points.

Hinders

If it sounds easy at this point, consider that both players (or even three or four) are trying to control the same 800 square-foot space. This often results in *a hinder.* The most commonly occurring hinders are events that interfere with a player's opportunity to have a clean shot at the ball. They include *accidental hinders,* (in which case the point is replayed), an *obstruction* or *avoidable hinder* (where the rally is forfeited), *player hinders* (hitting one's opponent "on the fly" with a ball on its way to the front wall), *court hinders* (the ball hitting some object on the court other than the walls, ceiling or floor), *body contact* (players colliding during a rally), *screen* (when vision is obscured), and a *backswing hinder* (when the opponent interferes with the space needed for a backswing). The avoidable hinder rule is used mostly in tournament play, when a referee is assigned. In most situations when recreational players call a hinder they simply play the point over. They do so to avoid squabbling and delays.

A *safety holdup* is when a player about to execute a swing holds up or stops the swing or movement toward the ball to avoid hitting the opponent with the ball or racquet.

During tournament play, these calls for blocks or hinders are left to the judgment of the referee; in most regular play, it is up to the players to decide. Even in the presence of a referee, the integrity of players is often challenged. For example, when the referee calls a point on a skipped shot, the ethical person will call the correct play (the unethical person will, of course, take the point).

Checklist for Hinders

1. Avoidable hinders (result in loss of point or serve)
   - Failure to move
   - Stroke interference
   - Blocking
   - Moving into the ball
   - Pushing
   - Intentional distractions
   - View obstruction
   - Wetting the ball
   - Apparel or equipment loss
2. Hinders (replay rally)
   - Court hinders
   - Ball hits opponent on return to wall
   - Body contact
   - Screen ball
   - Backswing hinder
   - Safety holdup
   - Other interferences

In the absence of a referee, all calls are completely up to the players; if there are any questions on a close play—*play it again.* The game is for the players' enjoyment—the challenge, the continuous movement, and the camaraderie of competitors—not for haggling over every call. Be honest with yourself and your partner on all physical action calls and rely on your opponent's reciprocal attitude. No point is worth risking injury to either player, so if a possible safety problem is anticipated, hold up that shot; when your opponent claims a safety holdup, be thankful and happily play it again. Always avoid hitting the other player(s) with the ball or the racquet.

Use the *golden rule of good judgment:* Respect the safety of other players as you would have them respect your own safety.

It is the responsibility of each player to avoid interfering with the opponent's fair chance to see and return the ball. It is also essential to move so that the opponent can go straight and directly to the ball and be allowed an unobstructed view of the play.

Avoidable hinders occur when one player fails to allow the other player full freedom to play a shot. The result of an avoidable hinder is side out or loss of point. Avoidable hinders include failure to move, stroke interference, blocking, moving into the ball, pushing, intentional distractions, and wetting the ball. It is the responsibility of the referee to call avoidable hinders. In the absence of a referee, players usually ignore this rule; an action that may lead to accidents.

Checklist of Safety Tips

1. Always know the location of the ball and other players.
2. Avoid contact with other players.
3. Be in control of the entire swing.
4. Do not take extra shots after play has ended.
5. Always knock and wait before entering a court.
6. Be sure wrist thongs are secure, and always wear protective eyewear.
7. Have a safety first—points second—attitude.

Safety Tips

Learn to avoid the type of play that leads to dangerous situations by always knowing the location of the ball and the other players on the court and by giving opponents their rightful opportunity to play each shot unobstructed.

Avoid contact with other players. If your opponent is between you and the ball, call a hinder. It is not necessary to crash into a player in order to call a hinder.

Do not swing wildly. Be in control of your follow-through.

Do not take extra shots after the point is ended, as players often relax after a rally and are vulnerable to injury at this time.

Always knock on the door and wait until it is clear before entering a court. An open door can be a hazard during a rally.

Be sure wrist thongs are secure and wear protective eyewear and protect yourself by being aware of the location of the ball and all players while on the court.

If you have an attitude of safety first—points second, racquetball can be a safe and enjoyable game.

Doubles Play

While singles play offers the most challenge to one's individual skills and can be a true test of conditioning levels, doubles and "cutthroat" are popular alternatives for physical education classes and crowded clubs. With three or four people in the same confined area, court safety becomes an increasingly important factor and the usual result is an increase in the number of hinders.

In doubles, the court is twice as crowded as in singles, making it necessary to be extra careful and more safety conscious. This means keeping aware of the position of three other bodies, not taking shots when the ball is close to another player, and calling a hinder when an opponent is in your path or in the way of your follow through (mainly, it means using good common sense).

Starting position for doubles

Server (1a) may stand anywhere in service zone.

Server's partner (1b) may stand in either service box (shaded areas).

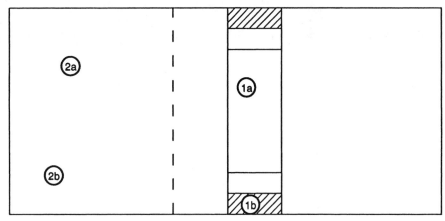

1 = serving team   2 = receiving team

Rule Differences for Doubles

In doubles play, there are only a few rule differences. First, the obvious: four players, two teams. The general flow of play is the same as in singles, except the teams instead of the players alternate hitting the ball. Either member of a team may hit the ball on that team's turn.

The major differences are in the manner of serve. The server still must stay within the confines of the service zone. The server's partner must remain standing in either service box, with his or her back against the wall, until the serve passes the short line. The two service boxes are located near the wall in the service zone. Violation of this rule results in loss of that service.

Also, if the server's partner enters the safety zone (the first five feet behind the service zone) before the ball passes the short line, the server loses the service. A served ball that hits the doubles partner while in the doubles box results in a fault serve. If the server's partner is hit by a serve that has already bounced, it would be considered a short serve (which is a fault serve).

A team retains the service until both players of that team have lost their service (hand), except on the opening serve of each game when the team that serves first gets only one hand; in that case only one partner serves. The order of serve must remain consistent during the entire game or the offending team loses service.

A ball that hits a player's partner results in a loss of point or service, but a ball that hits an opponent on its way to the wall is a hinder so that point is replayed unless the ball obviously didn't have enough velocity or direction to reach the front wall. In that case, the player who hit the ball loses the rally.

Nonofficial Types of Games

Cutthroat

This game is played with three players. There are two versions of cutthroat play: The server plays against a team of the other two opponents, or two

Checklist for Doubles Rule Differences

1. Teams consist of two players.
2. Either team member may hit the ball on that team's turn.
3. The server's partner must stay in the service box until the ball crosses the short line.
4. A team retains service until both members lose the serve, except on the first serve of each game.
5. The serving order must remain consistent.
6. The receiving team must observe the safety zone.
7. A ball that hits a player's partner results in loss of the serve or the point.
8. A ball on its way to the wall that hits a member of the opposition is a hinder, unless the ball obviously didn't have enough velocity or direction to reach the front wall. In that case, the player who hit the ball loses the rally.

players play singles with the third player on the back wall. The order of service is determined before the game begins, either by lagging for the short line (from a position near the back wall, each player hits the ball to the front wall; the player whose ball bounces back closest to the short line serves first) or by the flip of a coin.

In the first style of cutthroat (two against one), each time the service changes the teams alternate so that one player is playing against a team of two players. A player who loses the serve takes the place of the person who will serve next. This ensures the alternation of receivers so that one player is not serving to the same person's backhand for the entire game.

In the second style (third person out), two opponents play singles while the third player, who is not involved in the rally, stays along the back wall, shifting position as necessary in order to stay out of the way of the players and the ball. The player who loses the rally goes to the back wall, and the back-wall player takes the receiving position. The server either scores a point and retains the serve or loses the rally and becomes the back-wall person. A receiver who wins a rally becomes the server; the back-wall person will always become the receiver. Only the server can score, and the first player to score 15 points is the winner. Since the court is more crowded than in singles, the same extra safety precautions should be taken as in doubles.

Multi-Bounce

This is a game for children eight years old and under, but may be used by the physically handicapped, those people who are injured, the elderly, or as a drill for beginners.

After a serve puts the ball in play, the ball may bounce as many times as the receiver wishes, as long as it doesn't rebound from the back wall in front of the

Starting positions for cutthroat

a. Two against one: (1) serves first, (2) serves next, (3) serves next, (1) serves again.

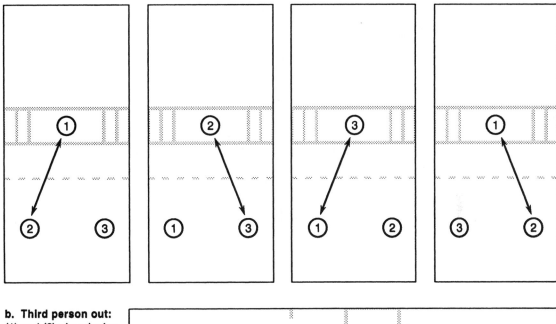

b. Third person out:
(1) and (2) play singles.
(3) remains against
wall out of play,
shifting position to
stay out of way, until
(1) loses serve and
replaces (3).
(3) replaces (2).
(2) replaces (1).

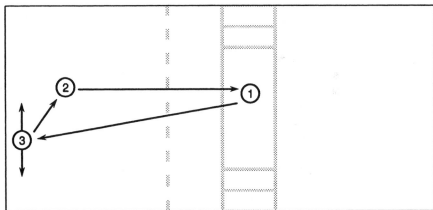

short line on its way to the front wall. (An exception is when the ball bounces off of the back wall directly on the fly. In this situation, the player may cross the short line to play the shot.)

Two Bounce

This is a higher-level game than no bounce; here, the player can let the ball bounce twice before it must be hit instead of the customary one bounce. Three bounces would result in the loss of the serve or the point.

This game is also recommended for youngsters, the handicapped, the elderly, mismatched players, and a drill for beginners.

Backhand Only

The rules of this game are the same as normal singles rules, except a player can only win a point or service by using a backhand shot. The backhand should be used on all serves and strokes. Forehand shots may be used to keep the ball in play, but points or service may not be gained from them. This is a good drill for players with weak backhands, or forehand-oriented sluggers who refuse to use their backhand. It is also used when players are mismatched. The better player can play backhand only, while the poorer player is allowed to use both forehand and backhand.

Ping-Pong Racquetball

Here is a game that utilizes table-tennis scoring. Each server gets five serves before yielding the serve. Either player can score on any point.

Both Score Racquetball

The Women's Professional Racquetball Tour followed this style of play during the early 1980s. It allows either person to score a point on every serve and the winner must win by 2 points. This places the emphasis of a close game at the end of the game and offers more spectator interest when the score is tied at 14 and either player can score. The server has the advantage by being able to serve for game control. In this game, the receiver is rewarded for a good return by winning both the point and the serve.

Warming Up Before Playing

Before beginning any athletic activity, it is essential to *warm up* the body in order to be able to play more efficiently and to reduce the chances of injury. Warming up stretches the muscles and tendons and forces muscle contractions, which get the body ready for the practice session or the game.

Start with a general body warm up of jogging or riding a stationary bicycle. This gets the blood flowing and increases the heart rate. Stretch the muscles and tendons that will be used during the activity. See Chapter 16 for a complete description of the exercises.

Before playing, it is recommended that a player stretch:

■ The hamstring muscles (the back of the thigh)
■ The quadriceps muscles (the front of the thigh)
■ The calf muscles and the Achilles tendons
■ The trunk muscles

Checklist for Nonofficial Games

1. Cutthroat is played with three players.
2. No bounce and two bounce are for younger, beginners or less-physically able players.
3. Backhand only is designed to improve the skill of the player with a weak backhand.
4. Ping-pong and both score provide alternate ways of scoring with nearly the same rules.

- The triceps (the back of the upper arm)
- The shoulder muscles

Each stretch should be done slowly and should be held for a minimum of 20 to 30 seconds without bouncing.

After stretching, hit the ball slowly using both forehand and backhand strokes and practice various shots. If a partner is available, start a slow rally, practicing each of your shots and hitting harder as your body warms up to the game.

Summary

1. The basic rule of racquetball is that players alternate hitting the ball to the front wall before it hits the floor a second time and only the server may score.
2. Play begins when one player, the server, puts the ball in play from inside the service area.
3. If the server wins a rally, a point is scored. If the receiver wins a rally, he or she gains the service.
4. The proper use of hinders plays an important role in the safety of the game.
5. Safety first should be a major concern of every player.
6. Doubles is played with teams of two players each.
7. There are a variety of alternate rules and games that can be enjoyed on the same racquetball court.

3

The Forehand

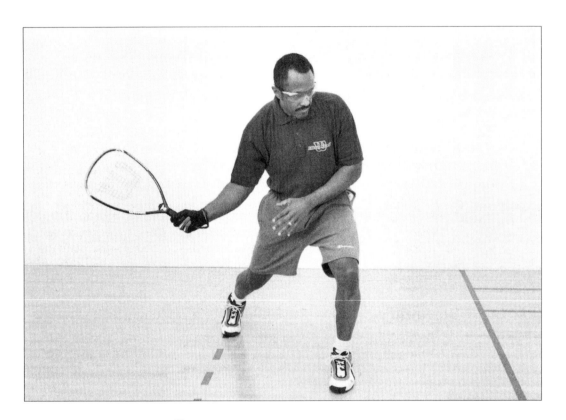

Outline

There is nothing mystical or magical about learning to play good, solid, consistent racquetball. The game is built around basic fundamentals; all of the wonderful, exciting shots people see and envy are either a forehand or a backhand placed at a specific area on the walls. Instead of trying to develop a myriad of fancy shots, it is more important to spend most of your practice time developing smooth, sound strokes and using them as a foundation to reach a consistent level of play.

The easiest way to understand the forehand shot is to break it down into specific segments, analyze each segment, and put them all together for a terrific end result: a solid forehand.

The Forehand Grip

Do not overlook this very important aspect of play. A *proper grip* is the first step in developing a consistent stroke.

In order to learn the proper forehand grip, one should imagine shaking hands with the racquet with the strings facing the walls, not the floor or ceiling. Place the "V" of your hand (where the thumb and index finger meet) on the top ridge of the handle. The middle and ring fingers should make contact lightly with the fleshy part of the lower thumb. This grip enables you to maintain a vertical hitting surface at the point of contact with the ball.

One way to check for correct grip is to swing the racquet face into the palm of your other hand. If the grip is correct, only the strings will strike the palm of

Proper grip

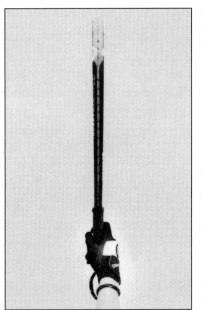 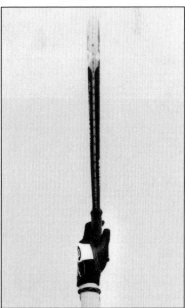

a. Right hand (from front)   **b. Left hand (from front)**

the hand. If, however, the grip has strayed to one side or the other, part of the frame will make contact with the hand (a very painful mistake!).

A common question is whether to hold the racquet high on the handle or down near the butt. The best answer is to hold the racquet wherever it feels most comfortable, keeping in mind the following guidelines:

1. Holding the racquet high on the handle will impede your wrist snap. This will be evident if the handle butt hits your wrist during the swing.

2. Holding the racquet near the end, so your little finger is off of the handle, will cause loss of control.

3. The style of your game should determine where to grip the handle: For more control, grip higher on the handle; for more power and wrist snap, grip the handle closer to the butt. This will provide more "whip" to your shots.

It is important to grip the racquet with fingers relaxed and slightly spread. Avoid taking a hammer grip or choke hold on the handle—racquetball is supposed to be fun, not preparation for hand-to-hand combat. Clamping down too

Improper Grips

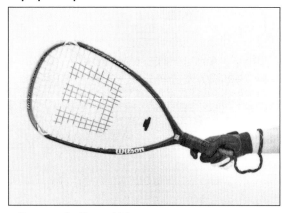

a. Proper grip (from side)

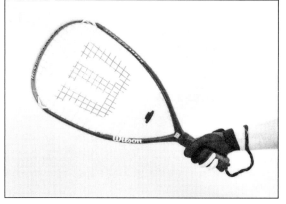

b. Hammer grip

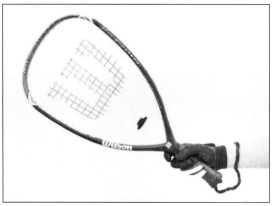

c. Choked up on handle

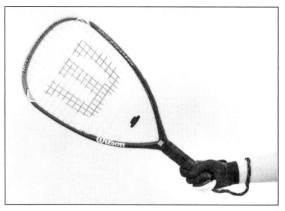

d. Too low on handle

Checklist for the Forehand Grip

1. Imagine shaking hands with the racquet.
2. Place the "V" of your hand on the top ridge of the handle.
3. The middle and ring fingers should make contact lightly with the fleshy part of the lower thumb.
4. The grip should be relaxed.

hard will tense and tire arm muscles, causing shots to stray off of the strings in various unplanned directions.

The Racquet-Ready Position

It is important to keep the racquet above waist level, positioned at the center of the body ready to move in any direction. With the racquet in this *ready position* (see illustration below), the transition to the backswing for both the forehand and the backhand will be quicker and more efficient.

Holding the racquet below waist level at one's side (a common error) is less efficient, because it slows down reaction time by increasing how long it takes to get into the backswing position, which means less power and accuracy.

Racquet-Ready Position

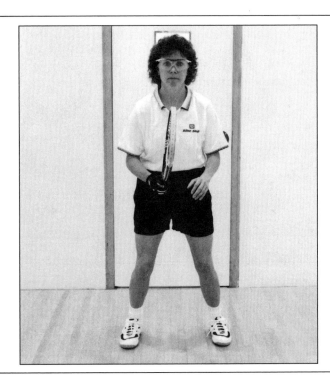

The Forehand Backswing

Having played baseball or softball can be a big help in learning the forehand. The motion used in swinging a bat is basically the same as that of swinging a racquetball racquet.

Let's compare the two swings: When at bat, do you stand with the front of your body facing the pitcher? No!! You stand sideways, with one shoulder facing the pitcher in order to be able to step into the ball, pivot your hips, and swing the bat through to the other side of your body, hitting the ball in the process. Racquetball utilizes the same principle: When a ball is hit to your forehand side, pivot your feet and turn to face that same-side wall. Keeping your knees slightly bent will make it easier to pivot and to get into good hitting position.

The second comparison is in preparing to swing a bat. Do you hold the bat down at your waist or resting on your shoulder? The bat should be held high and away from your body so no time is wasted beginning the swing. A racquetball swing is similar in that the racquet is raised to the pose one would use if trying to show-off the biceps muscle (your upper arm bone parallel to the floor), pointing the top edge of the racquet toward the ceiling. This position enables you to take a full swing and hit the ball with adequate

The racquetball swing and the swing in baseball or softball have much in common.

Ready stance:

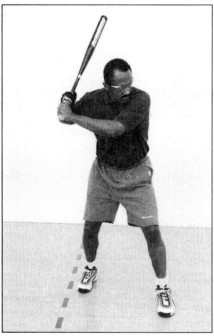

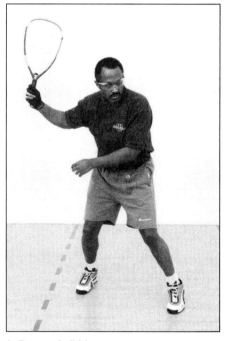

a. Softball hitter   **b. Racquetball hitter**

Point of contact:

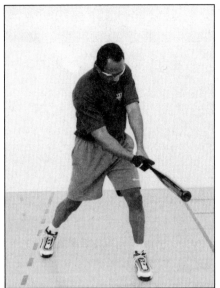 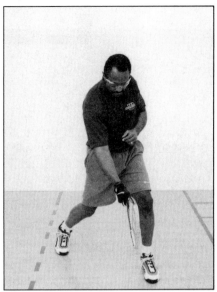

| c. Softball hitter | d. Racquetball hitter |

Follow-through:

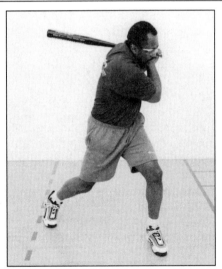 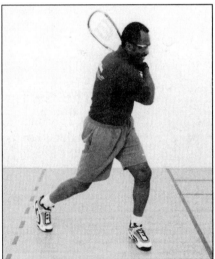

| e. Softball hitter | f. Racquetball hitter |

power. Shortening the backswing will cause you to push the ball to the wall. It is this pushing motion that is the cause of many shoulder and elbow injuries. A full and properly executed backswing is important to both your game and your health.

Checklist for the Forehand Backswing

1. From the ready position, pivot until you are facing the side wall on your forehand side.
2. Your upper arm bone should be parallel to the floor.
3. Point the top edge of the racquet at the ceiling.
4. Keep your knees slightly bent.
5. Keep your eyes on the ball and your head down.

Checklist for the Forehand Swing

1. The swing begins with the forward motion of the arm holding the racquet.
2. As the swing begins, bend your wrist and lower the racquet from its backswing position.
3. The top end of the racquet points to the back wall.
4. The butt of the handle faces the front wall.
5. After meeting requirements 3 and 4 above, snap the wrist and bring the racquet strings through the ball, arms extended away from the body.
6. Make your swing as level as possible.

The Swing

Let's continue with our baseball/racquetball analogy. When swinging a bat, do you hit down on the ball or try to be like Bo Jackson and swing up for a home run? Consistency comes from swinging as levelly as possible and trying to hit a line drive every time. This requires swinging the bat away and to the side of the body, with the hands and arms fully extended.

The *racquetball swing* begins with a forward motion of the arm holding the racquet. As you begin this forward movement, bend your wrist back, lowering the racquet from its backswing position, so that the top end of the racquet is pointing toward the back wall and the butt of the handle is facing the front wall. As soon as these two points of reference are met, snap your wrist and bring the racquet strings through the ball. Your arm should be fully extended away from your body at the very moment contact with the ball is made just like when hitting a line drive in baseball.

Point of Contact

Think of an imaginary line extending from the top of the head, down the middle of the face, and continuing down the middle of the body. This imaginary

Close-up of the Forehand Swing

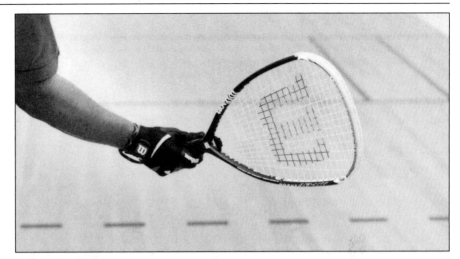

a. Wrist before contact

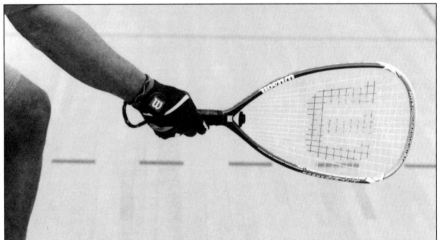

b. Wrist at point of contact

line divides the body into two equal halves. Regarding the position of the ball in relation to this line, the point of contact should be *in front of this line.* The space between the middle of the body and front foot is the *contact area.* Making contact with the ball in front of this midline allows the forward momentum of the body and arm to swing smoothly into the ball. This will result in more power and consistency than when the contact point is in the area behind the midline.

The height at which contact should be made depends on the type of shot selected, but the general area is between the calf and the middle of the thigh. The ball should be hit after it has reached its highest point and is on its way down. A natural instinct is to be impatient and rush forward to hit the ball, instead of waiting to let it drop into the desired contact zone.

Point of contact

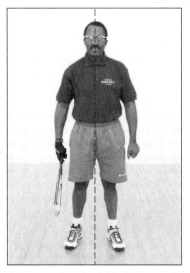
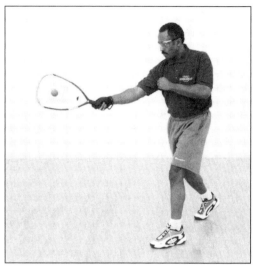

Contact point should be in front of the imaginary vertical line.

Incorrect: Contact point too high

Point of contact: Ball is hit on downward flight after reaching highest point (apex)

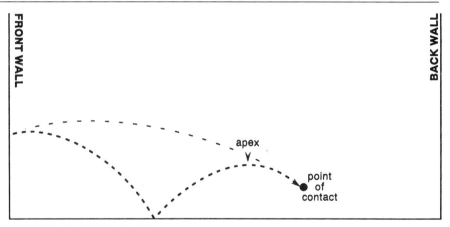

Follow-Through

After contact, it is imperative to complete the swing. A very common error occurs when players stop the swing and don't follow through. This can result in three problems: injuries, inconsistent shots, and loss of power.

The *injuries* that result from this practice are "tennis elbow" and tendonitis of the shoulder joint. A tremendous amount of force and racquet speed are created by taking a full backswing and stepping into the point of contact. To abruptly stop all that forward momentum places a great amount of stress on the elbow and shoulder joints.

Inconsistent shots result when one doesn't realize that *follow-through* is the main factor in determining the direction or path the ball travels. Also, the lack

Follow-through

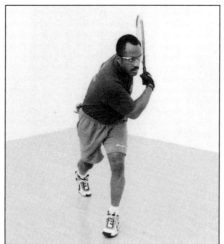

a. Correct

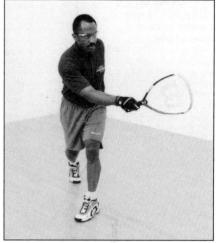

b. Incorrect: Stopping short

✓   *Checklist for the Forehand Follow-Through*

1. Complete the swing after making contact with the ball.
2. A smooth follow-through determines the direction of the shot.
3. After hitting the ball, the racquet should continue in its path unimpeded.
4. The swing ends when the racquet comes to rest in the area behind the nonhitting shoulder.

of a smooth follow through leads to loss of power—shots made without adequate velocity stray to undesirable spots on the walls.

The follow through should allow the racquet to swing unimpeded until it comes to rest somewhere in the area behind the non-hitting shoulder.

Nonhitting Arm

One of the most difficult problems of the forehand swing is dealing with *hitting across your body.* There is an arm and a leg in front of your body that can get in the way of the shot.

One solution is to keep the *nonhitting arm* down by your side, allowing forward momentum to swing it away from the shot. Avoid tucking it into your body, as this will inhibit a smooth follow through. Also, do not hold or touch the racquet with the free hand—using the nonhitting hand to hold the racquet will restrict the backswing, cutting down on the available power.

Incorrect use of non-hitting arm by tucking it under other arm or next to body

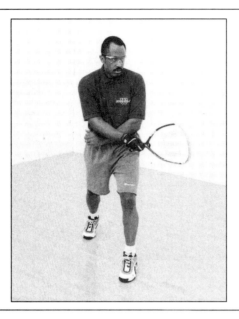

Using the Lower Body

The *legs and hips* also combine with the arm and wrist to add power to the shot. Shifting weight from the back to the front foot supplies that extra power.

Assume a stance sideways to the ball, knees slightly bent, with the back foot (the foot closest to the back wall) solidly planted. From this position, stride diagonally toward the ball and in the direction of the swing. This striding motion will allow use of the entire body, while helping to maintain good balance.

Stepping directly toward the side wall, instead of diagonally, makes it difficult to get weight and momentum into the swing, forcing the player to use only the arm to propel the ball. Stepping directly toward the front wall causes a loss of balance after the swing by forcing the body's weight backward, taking momentum in a direction away from the rally instead of toward a good court position.

As the front leg strides toward the point of contact, the back knee should begin to bend and the back leg should be kept in contact with the floor, providing a solid base from which to pivot. The toe should remain in contact with the floor. Bending the back knee enables the player to lower the center of gravity, so the racquet can swing through the ball and parallel to the floor.

As the weight shifts from the back foot to the front, the hips also pivot to deliver more power. At this point, concentrate on driving your right buttock into each shot. If you are left-handed, use the left buttock.

Even though the point of contact is below the waist, do not lower your upper body by bending at the waist; always bend at the knees. This will keep your upper body erect and your weight over your base, permitting a level swing. Bending at the waist will cause the racquet face to drop from the desired parallel position, making you hit downward, skipping the ball into the floor.

Lower body stride

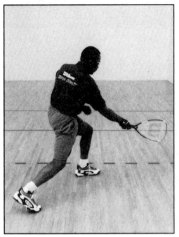 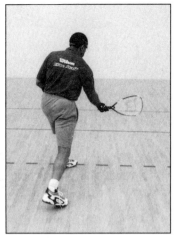 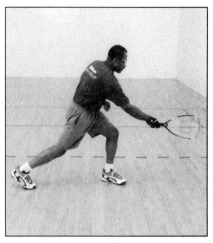

| **a. Correct** | b. Incorrect to front wall | c. Incorrect to side wall |

Bending to meet ball

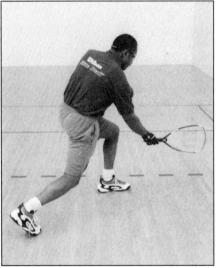 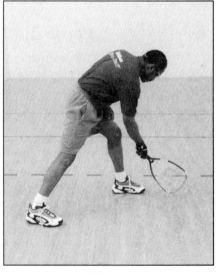

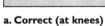

a. Correct (at knees)   b. Incorrect (at waist)

This is an appropriate place to further explain the height of the point of contact. If you have enough time to properly set up for a shot, the ideal contact point is somewhere in the area between the calf and the knee, provided that the upper body has been lowered by the player bending at the knees.

When attempting to hit a kill shot, opt for making contact with the ball at calf level; for a pass shot, knee-high contact should be adequate. (See Chapter 7 for a complete discussion of kill and pass shots.)

Checklist for Using the Lower Body

1. Stand sideways to the ball, facing the side wall.
2. Have the knees slightly bent, back foot solidly planted.
3. Stride diagonally toward the ball.
4. Bend the back knee and pivot on the back toe.
5. Keep your upper body erect.
6. Concentrate on driving the buttock into the ball.
7. Wait for the ball to drop into the desired contact zone.

Eye Focus

Performing all of the steps of the swing perfectly loses its value unless your *eyes remain focused* on the ball until after the moment of contact.

Often a player will miss an easy set up because, at the last moment before contact, he or she lifts the head to see where to hit the ball instead of focusing only on the ball. A good catch-phrase to help remember this is "Keep your eyes on the ball, instead of the wall."

Forehand Advice

This chapter described the goals for a strong forehand, though in reality, the classic shot may be very difficult to execute in a fast-paced game. The ball travels at high speeds and there is often not enough time to hit a picture-perfect shot. In order to be able to play a consistent game, it is important to develop a base of skills built on solid fundamentals. Try to take a full swing through the ball whenever possible. Power will mask flaws and mistakes; go for power first, control second.

Common Forehand Errors

1. *Improper grip*—Since the desired point of contact should be below waist level, a grip error could allow the strings to face the floor at the point of contact, resulting in a skipped shot. Or if your grip allows the racquet head to face upward, the result will be balls hitting on the front wall higher than planned.

2. *Pushing the ball*—A short backswing without a proper follow-through is known as a *wimp shot* and will cut power and impede accuracy. Think "power first, control second." Power can mask mistakes, and allows the player more margin for error. A powerfully hit shot forces the opponent to react faster and does not need to be quite as accurate as a slower, control-oriented shot. The short, punching stroke is an attempt to stress accuracy by aiming the ball; this is a bad habit that can hinder a person's chance to develop into a complete player.

    Racquetball is a fast, aggressive sport. That's what makes it such a popular and enjoyable activity. Get out on the court and hit the ball as hard as

Eye focus

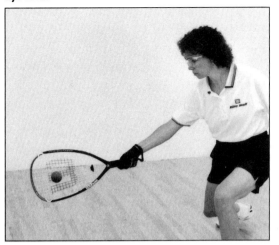 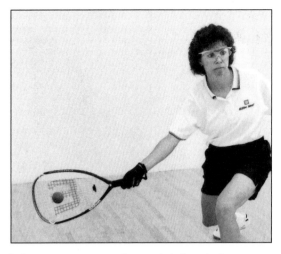

a. Correct: at point of contact with ball   **b. Incorrect: eyes away from point of contact**

Full forehand sequence

From side:

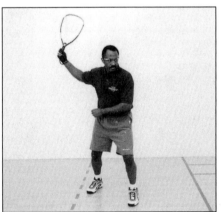 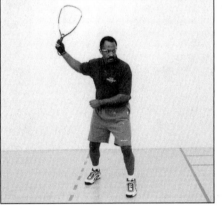

a. Backswing   **b. Swing**

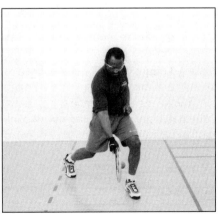 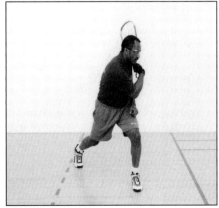

c. Contact   **d. Follow-through**

Full forehand sequence

From above:

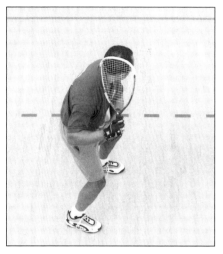

e. Backswing

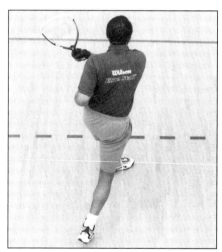

f. Swing

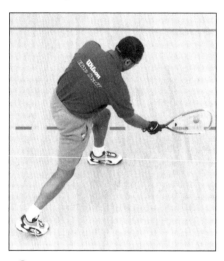

g. Contact

h. Follow-through

you possibly can *with good form,* getting a good workout, and having a lot of fun doing it. Take a full swing!

3. *Too close for comfort*—Letting the ball get too close to the body results in a restricted swing and can cause a player with a beautiful, smooth stroke to lose the rhythm of the swing and impede the follow through. This is what is known in racquetball circles as playing out of control. For maximum power, reach out for the ball away from your body, allowing full arm extension at the point of contact.

4. *Not using the legs*—Being lazy and failing to stress basic footwork and the fundamentals of body position result in using only the arm to provide power. This contributes to sore shoulders and elbows. It is important to position your legs so your body can face the side wall; then, with knees flexed, use your legs to drive forward into the ball.

> ✓   *Checklist for the Forehand*
>
> 1. Make sure that the "V" of the hand is at the top of the racquet's handle and that the racquet face is exactly perpendicular to the floor.
> 2. Face the side wall before getting ready to swing.
> 3. Take a full backswing with your racquet arm away from your body.
> 4. Take a diagonal stride toward the ball, using your legs to drive forward, and bend at your knees instead of your waist to position your body lower when making shots.
> 5. To help visualize your stroke, think of a baseball player hitting a line drive (with a flat stroke), not a golfer with a circular or pendulum-like swing.
> 6. Make sure your wrist is cocked until the last moment, then whip it through the ball. Do not punch, push, or aim the ball.
> 7. Make contact with the ball while it is on its downward flight, at a height between the calf and the knee, in front of the mid-line of your body, and even with your front foot.
> 8. Keep your head down and your eyes focused on the ball.
> 9. Keep the nonhitting arm down at your side.
> 10. Follow through on your swing completely, to the point behind your opposite shoulder.

5. *Impatience*—One of the most common errors that beginning and intermediate players make is to rush directly toward the ball and make contact near the highest point of its trajectory, instead of waiting for it to drop into the proper hitting zone (usually around knee or calf level).

Summary

1. For consistent forehand play, practice to develop a smooth, sound swing.
2. The grip is an important first step in the right direction. An improper grip will not permit a player to execute a proper swing.
3. A correct backswing is a necessary element of the swing, as it enables the player to take a full swing.
4. A level, full swing allows for maximum power and control.
5. Allowing the ball to drop into the contact zone and keeping your eyes focused on the ball until after it is hit is important for control.
6. Even after hitting the ball, the swing must continue unimpeded until the racquet completes its full arc and comes to rest behind the opposite shoulder.
7. The lower body provides proper body positioning and power by driving the hips into the swing.
8. Your ready position, pivot, backswing, forward movement, stride into the ball, level swing, eye focus, wrist snap, and follow-through must all be coordinated to make a complete forehand stroke.

4 *The Backhand*

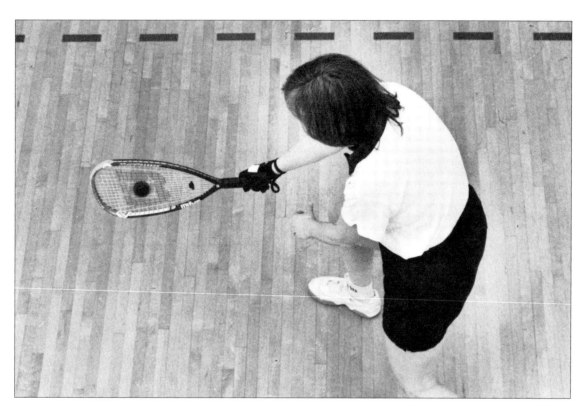

Outline

At most clinics and teaching camps, the number one concern of most players is hitting a stronger, more consistent backhand. Perhaps because the forehand motion is more commonly used in other activities, players have more confidence in their forehand swings. But the backhand is really not that difficult—you can have a better backhand if you follow these three simple rules:

1. Think shoulder
2. Take a full swing
3. Practice, practice, practice

The Backhand Grip

Whenever there is enough time to change the grip (which is almost always), switch to the *backhand grip.* This is accomplished by making a slight adjustment to the forehand grip. Beginning with the forehand grip, move the V made by the thumb and index finger from the top ridge of the racquet handle to the next ridge to the left (or to the right if you are left-handed), a slight rotation toward the thumb. This minor adjustment enables the racquet head to contact the ball on a level plane.

If the forehand grip is used for the backhand stroke, the strings, or face of the racquet, will be facing slightly toward the ceiling, causing the shots to lift in a slicing manner. By making this one-eighth of an inch rotation toward the thumb, the player may hit the ball more solidly and with more consistency.

Change from forehand grip to backhand grip

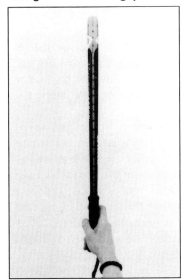

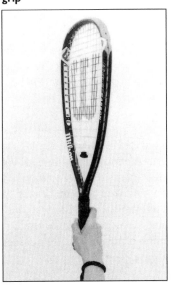

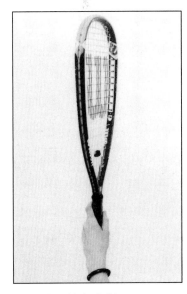

a. Forehand   **b. Change-over to backhand**   **c. Backhand grip (left)**

Checklist for the Backhand Grip

1. To change to the backhand grip from the forehand grip, move the V slightly toward your thumb.
2. Make this slight change with your racquet hand and fingers, not your other hand.
3. If time is not available to make this change, use the forehand grip and make the best of the situation.

Do not get into the bad habit of using the nonhitting hand to turn the racquet; let your racquet hand and fingers do it for you. The practice of using the nonhitting hand will inhibit your backhand backswing and lengthen the time it takes you to get the racquet into the backswing position. However, if you are positioned too near the front wall to have enough time to change the grip, go ahead and use whatever grip is available and make the best of the situation.

Racquet-Ready Position

The *racquet-ready position* is the same for the backhand stroke as for the forehand, since the player does not know to which side of the body the shot will be coming. The racquet should be held with only one hand, above waist level, at the center of the body.

The Backhand Backswing

The backhand stroke involves less wrist snap than the forehand, consequently much of the power comes from a full *backswing* that rotates the shoulders back and the racquet up and away from the body. This position sets the stage for a swing that provides the racquet head with a good deal of speed and momentum as it goes into the ball.

Learn to think of the racquet as an extension of your arm. Unlike the forehand, the backhand is not a wrist stroke. Do nothing with your wrist at this time.

Whenever attempting a backhand, always stand facing the side wall, in order to be positioned sideways to any ball returning from the front wall. From this position, extend your arm and racquet directly in front of you, so the top of the racquet is pointing at the side wall and the strings are facing the front and back walls. Next, rotate your elbow until the top edge of the racquet faces the backwall, forming a right angle (90 degrees). The strings should now be facing the side walls. Now, continue to move the racquet toward the back wall until your shoulder makes contact with your chin. Your shoulders should now be all the way around so that your chest is facing the back wall, but your head should still be facing the side wall so that you can keep eye contact with the ball. In

Backhand backswing

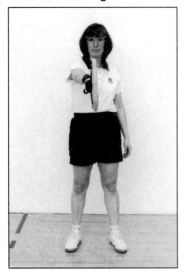 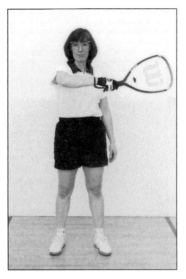 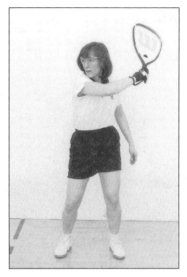

a. Extended arm and racquet   b. Elbow bent   c. Turn chest to back wall

---

✓ Checklist for the Backhand Backswing

1. Think of the racquet as extension of your arm.
2. While facing the side wall, your arm should be extended so the top of the racquet is pointing to the side wall.
3. Your elbow should be bent, forming a right angle.
4. The racquet should be moved back until your shoulder makes contact with your chin.
5. Your chest should be facing the back wall.
6. Your knees should be slightly bent.

order to execute this pivot, your knees must be bent, with your weight on the balls of your feet (otherwise, your hip will be locked and unable to pivot).

The Swing

Once the backswing has been completed, the racquet is ready to be brought into the ball (the *swing*). But if the backhand stroke is executed directly from the backswing, the ball will be hit into the floor; consequently, some adjustment is necessary.

Remembering the baseball swing, use your shoulder to lower the racquet while it is behind your body, then leading with the shoulder, pull the racquet

Backhand swing and point of contact

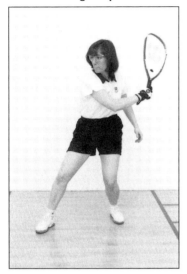

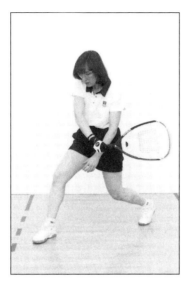

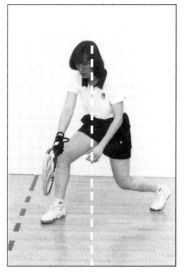

a. Drop racquet head

b. Shoulder leads

c. Point of contact is forward of the midline of your body (indicated by line)

✓ *Checklist for the Backhand Swing*

1. Use your shoulder to lower the racquet.
2. Use your shoulder to pull the racquet through the ball.
3. Your arm should be fully extended.
4. Keep a firm wrist during the swing.
5. Emphasize punching through the ball, by leading with your shoulder.

through the ball, out to the side. At the point of contact with the ball, your arm should be fully extended toward the side wall.

There is very little wrist motion in the backhand swing, a factor that causes problems for many players. Most people have heard that racquetball is a sport that emphasizes wrist action, which is true in the case of the forehand swing. But if the wrist is used in the same manner during the backhand, the ball will consistently be dumped directly into the ground. In other words, keep a firm wrist throughout the backswing and emphasize punching through the ball by leading with your shoulder.

The Point of Contact

Divide your body in half with the same imaginary perpendicular line that was used with the forehand swing. The striking area still should be forward of this

Checklist for the Point of Contact

1. The striking area should be forward of the midline of the body, even with the forward foot.
2. Your weight should be on your forward foot.
3. Contact the ball on its downward flight, at a height between the calf and the middle of the thigh.
4. Always keep your eyes focused on the ball.

midline, except that the backhand swing's *point of contact* is farther forward than that of the forehand.

It is crucial that you make contact with the ball while your weight is on the forward foot. Without benefit of an explosive wrist snap (as with the forehand), your weight must be forward, to allow the face of the racquet to properly complete the swing.

The height of the point of contact is the same as with the forehand, depending on court position and the type of shot selected. The basic contact area is still from mid-thigh to mid-calf.

As with the forehand, it is important to keep your eyes focused on the ball during all phases of the backhand.

Follow-Through

After making contact with the ball, keep a firm wrist and let the racquet continue unimpeded, in the most level and horizontal manner possible. At the end of the *follow-through,* the racquet should be pointing toward the opposite side wall, not at the ceiling or the floor.

Just as in the follow through of the forehand swing, failing to allow the racquet to finish its full swing may result in shoulder and elbow injuries. Many nagging physical problems can be avoided by allowing the entire body to absorb the force of the swing, not only the elbow and the shoulder.

Checklist for Backhand Follow-Through

1. Keep a firm wrist.
2. After making contact with the ball, let the racquet continue on its arc unimpeded.
3. At the end of the follow-through, the racquet should be pointing at the opposite side wall.
4. As with the forehand swing, stopping the follow through prematurely can result in shoulder and elbow injuries.

Follow-through

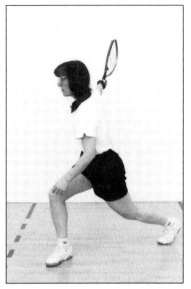 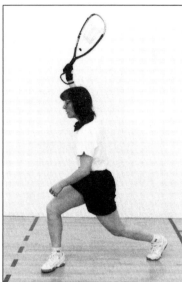

a. Correct   **b. Racquet pointing up**

**Incorrect:
b, c, and d**

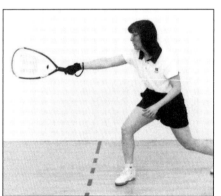 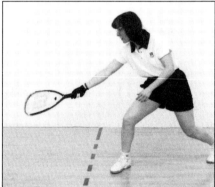

c. Racquet pointing to front wall   **d. Racquet pointing down**

Nonhitting Arm

Since the backhand is mainly a shoulder stroke, it is important to allow the shoulder a full, unrestricted rotation. In order for this to happen, the *nonhitting arm* must be kept out of the way of the swing. Some players take the racquet back with two hands, while others keep their nonhitting arm tucked against the chest. Both of these practices restrict the backward movement of the shoulders that is necessary during the backswing. Players not taking a full backswing will be forever doomed to a wimpy, powerless backhand *push shot.*

Keep the nonhitting hand and arm relaxed and slightly bent at your side, allowing it to help balance your body.

Incorrect uses of nonhitting arm

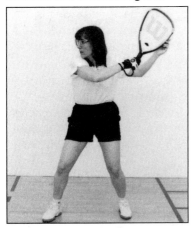
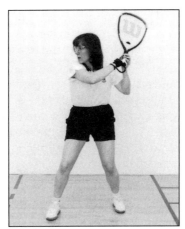
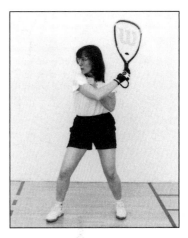

a. Two hands on racquet	**b. Two hands on racquet**	**c. Arm tucked**

Using the Lower Body

Your *legs and hips* play as important a role in the backhand as they do in the forehand. By shifting the main part of your weight from your back foot to your front, you create forward momentum. This forward momentum supplies the backhand with a large part of its power.

When preparing to make a backhand swing, always try to stand like a batter awaiting a pitch and face the side wall before making that diagonal, forward stride with your front foot. This forward step and the resulting weight shift will add that necessary momentum.

In the backhand, the legs are used in a manner similar to the forehand. Plant your back foot, stride diagonally into the shot, bend your knees to lower your trunk, drive the rear buttock into the shot, and use your legs for maximum power and consistency.

 Checklist for Using the Lower Body

1. Plant your back foot to give a solid base.
2. Stride diagonally into the shot.
3. Bend your back knee to allow your body to get a lower position for the shot.
4. Lower your center of gravity by bending at the knees, not at the waist.
5. Drive the buttocks into the shot.
6. Keep your upper body erect.
7. Make contact with the ball at a point even with your front foot.
8. Use your legs for maximum power and consistency.

Common Errors in the Backhand

1. *Improper grip*—The most common grip error in the backhand swing is keeping a forehand grip. Not changing your grip to the recommended backhand grip and instead trying to use one, all-purpose grip will result in sliced shots and balls hit too high on the front wall.

2. *Wrist flick*—Trying to use the wrist to flick at shots with the backhand swing, because of the myth that the sport is "all wrist," results in weak shots. Avoid cocking your wrist during the backswing because it promotes a pendulum swing and is an extra movement that may cause timing problems. Instead, keep a firm wrist during the entire stroke, using the racquet as an extension of your arm.

3. *Incomplete backswing*—Some players do not utilize a full backswing because they try to overemphasize accuracy or because the proper backswing stroke feels awkward at first. Without pulling the racquet back and reaching the full backswing position, a player will never know the joy of hearing the ball "pop" when it hits the front wall on a backhand shot. An incomplete backswing causes a short, powerless stroke and could result in a shoulder or elbow injury.

4. *Too close for comfort*—Hitting the ball when it is too close to the body is another common mistake. As with the forehand, the ball must be kept away from the body, allowing a full-arm extension and a full swing. Hitting the ball while it is close to the body promotes pushing shots instead of hitting them with a full, unrestricted stroke.

Backhand stride

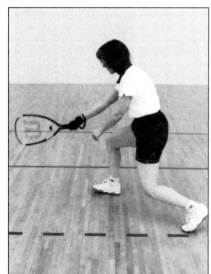 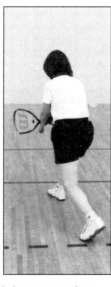 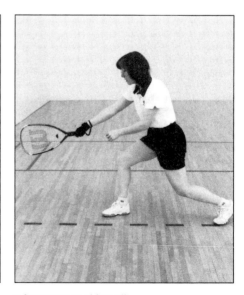

a. Correct

b. Incorrect to front wall

c. Incorrect to side wall

From side: Full backhand sequence

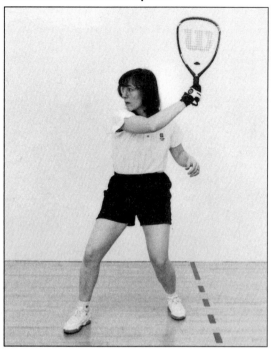

a. Backswing

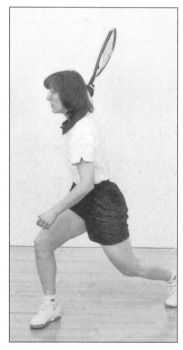

b. Beginning of swing

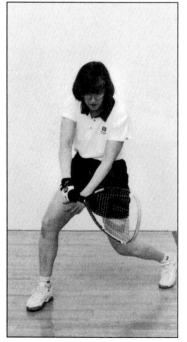

c. Swing

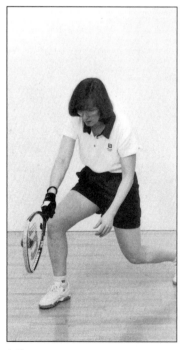

d. Contact

e. Follow-through

From above: Full backhand sequence

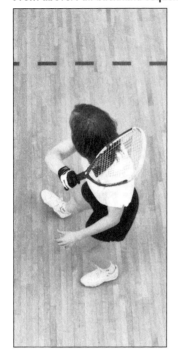

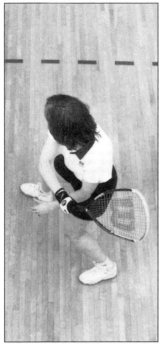

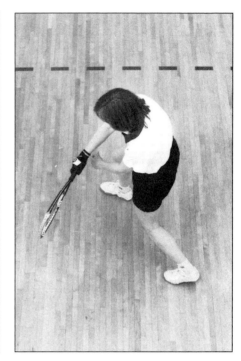

f. Backswing   g. Beginning of swing   h. Swing

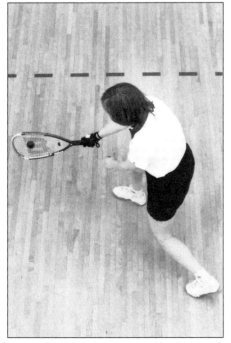

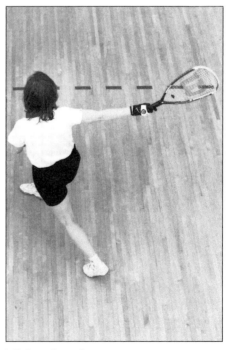

i. Contact   j. Follow through

Checklist for the Backhand

1. Rotate the grip one-eighth turn toward the thumb to provide a vertical hitting surface.
2. Face the side wall.
3. Rotate your shoulders back until your chest is facing the back wall and your head is facing the side wall so you can keep your eye on the ball.
4. Drop the racquet behind your body and swing out to the side, arm and racquet extended.
5. Take a long, diagonal stride into the shot.
6. Begin the swing by driving your shoulder into the ball, keeping a firm wrist (do not employ a wrist snap).
7. The point of contact should be even with your front foot and between the calf and the middle of the thigh.
8. Keep your head down and your eyes on the ball.
9. Follow through the entire swing—do not stop its momentum or rhythm.

Summary

1. Improving one's backhand is a major concern of many players.
2. Guidelines to improving one's backhand are (1) think shoulders, (2) take a full swing, and (3) practice, practice, practice.
3. A minor adjustment from the forehand grip is necessary to allow for a level backhand swing.
4. The backswing sets the stage for a swing that provides racquet speed and momentum into the ball.
5. The shoulder is used to lower the racquet from the backswing position and start the momentum into the ball.
6. Your wrist should remain stiff during the backswing.
7. Allow the ball to drop into the desired hitting zone and make contact when the ball is even with your front foot.
8. Follow-through is as important in the backhand as it is in the forehand stroke.
9. Your eyes must be focused on the ball until after the moment of contact.
10. Your legs and hips provide power and momentum as you stride into the ball.
11. To make a complete backhand stroke, the following actions must be coordinated: (1) being in the ready position, (2) pivoting so that your chest faces the back wall, (3) moving your shoulder forward so that it is begins the forward momentum, (4) striding into the ball, (5) making a level swing while keeping your eyes focused on the ball, and (6) completing an uninhibited follow-through.

5

Court Coverage and Doubles Play

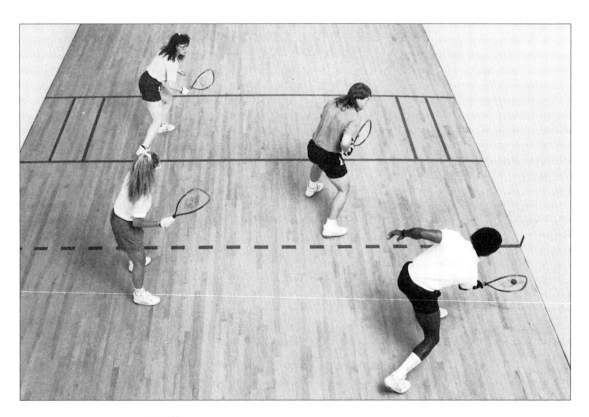

Outline

Where you play on the court and how you move to the ball are essential fundamentals of the game of racquetball. Not only must the body be ready to move and hit, it must be in the best position to defend the court.

The Ready Position

Every sport that requires quick movement begins with the player in a *ready position*. The ready position is similar for a racquetball player, a defensive back in football, an infielder in baseball, or a tennis or badminton player.

When a player is in the ready position, we should find:

- Feet placed at shoulder width or slightly wider, allowing the player to execute quick lateral movements
- Knees slightly bent, allowing for quick movement in any direction
- Weight on the balls of the feet, helping prepare for quick movement
- Body bent slightly at the waist, putting the weight over the balls of the feet
- Head up, helping to see the entire court
- Racquet held above waist level in the center of the body and pointing upward, and elbows bent (allowing for quick rotation to either the forehand or backhand side)

The most common faults are:

- The body held too straight and stiff
- The player standing flat-footed, with too much weight toward the heels
- The racquet held too low

Any of these will reduce one's potential for quick movement.

Court Coverage

From the ready position, it is essential that *the player be able to move quickly, easily, and effectively in the direction the shot is hit.* As a player becomes more skilled and experienced, it will be possible to anticipate more accurately the spot where contact with the ball can best be made. Beginners often do a great

 Checklist for the Ready Position

1. The player's feet are placed at shoulder width or slightly wider.
2. The player's knees are slightly bent.
3. The player's weight is on the balls of the feet.
4. The player is bent slightly forward at the waist.
5. The player's head is up.
6. The racquet is held above waist level, elbows bent.

Step-together-step sequence

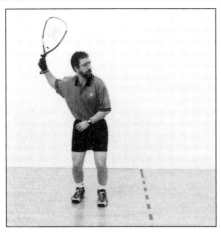

a. Feet together

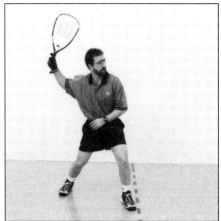

b. Step

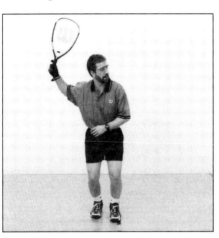

c. Feet together

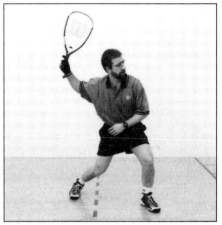

d. Step

deal of needless running as they chase the ball, while skilled players quickly see where the shot should be played and move to that spot.

Whenever possible the player should shuffle to the ball rather than running to it (sliding the feet without crossing the legs using the "step-together-step" footwork). This shuffling action keeps the body in a better position to step correctly into a shot. Of course, if covering a long distance, run to the ball as quickly as possible.

Stay on your toes whenever the ball is in play, maintaining the ready position with your feet in motion. Anticipate your opponent's shot as much as possible and move as the shot is being made. Too many players stand flat-footed and hope that the ball will bounce somewhere near them. Good players are constantly moving and anticipating where they think they can make the most effective shot and win the rally.

Checklist for Court Coverage

1. Use the step-together-step method and shuffle to the ball.
2. Stay on your toes, bouncing lightly, and maintain the ready position.
3. Hit and move! Hit and move!

As you wait for your opponent's shot, keep bouncing lightly on your toes so that you are always moving—this gives the greatest chance of reacting rapidly once the direction of the ball is observed. Then stop the bouncing, pivot your hips so that you face the side wall, and get to the ball. Remember, hit and move! Hit and move!

Concentration and Anticipation

Concentration plays a big role in *anticipation*. To win at racquetball you need to have your eyes, mind, and body totally focused on the ball. Your attitude should be one of persistent determination. Your eyes should never lose sight of the ball from the moment it's dropped for the serve until the rally is ended. Watching your opponent prepare to contact the ball allows you to anticipate the shot as it travels to the front wall. The sole exception to this practice is the moment an opponent is actually making contact with the ball. For added confidence in watching the ball at all times you should always wear protective eyewear when on the court.

By keeping your eyes on the ball you will be able to quickly determine a number of things about the shot that will aid in retrieving it. You will be able to tell whether an opponent's shot will be hit hard or soft, toward the ceiling (shoulder height), as a pass (waist height), or as a kill (calf height). You will also be able to tell the direction of the shot; how much time you have to set up for the return; and whether to run up, move back, or get to center court.

As soon as you determine the direction of the shot, decide whether to move right or left in response to it. Beginners usually wait until they see the ball rebound from the front wall, while advanced players are moving as the ball leaves the opponent's racquet.

This is a difficult skill to master while playing on the court. You will need to watch others playing so that you can concentrate on different types of strokes, tendencies, and shot placements. You should eventually be able to predict the shot and its direction before a player even hits the ball.

In addition to your eyes, you should have your mind and body focused on the current rally. The last thing you want to do is hit a shot and stand around. Be constantly moving, bouncing, looking for an edge, and ready to attack the shot by being in the best possible return position. A racquetball moves tremendously fast (ninety-plus miles per hour for the average player), so by being ready you'll be doing yourself a favor and giving yourself more time to react. Hit and move! Hit and move!

Center Court Position

In most sports, the player who controls the action will probably win the game. In hockey, a team must control the area near the goal. In tennis, a player must control the net. In racquetball, a player who wants to win must control the *center court.*

Since a racquetball court is twenty feet by forty feet, the exact center of the court is a spot ten feet from the side walls and twenty feet from the front wall. Controlling the exact center of the court is not what is meant by *center court control.* "Center court" is an oval area behind the short service line, extending to arm and racquet distance from either side wall.

This area is called *flowing center court.* While in this area you want to "flow" from side to side, depending on the location of your opponent. For example, if your opponent is about to hit a backhand from the deep left corner of the court, you should be on the left side of the oval, closest to your opponent's position. This places you in a position to cover a *down the line,* or *straight shot,* and you will still have time to reach a cross-court shot. When your opponent is about to hit the ball, always be in a position to cover the shot with the least travel time. In the above example, a straight shot has less distance to travel than a cross-court shot, so you should play to the left side of the court.

Whenever possible, be on the same side of center court toward which the opponent's shot is heading. In addition to covering the most direct return shot your opponent can hit, you also give the impression that you are ready and waiting for the expected shot. This often causes an alteration of your opponent's normal shot selection or game plan, which is an added advantage.

Center court position offers many advantages. It provides a player with an opportunity to attack with a variety of offensive shots—kill shots, pinch shots, and low pass shots—as well as being in position to reach more of the opponent's shots. (Offensive shots are covered in detail in Chapter 7.)

The ideal situation is to play in mid-court and keep your opponent in back court. Some advantages to this strategy are that your opponent will have to retrieve your shots from deep court and be forced to run around you to reach the ball, and your body might block your opponent's view of the ball for a brief moment.

When you are stuck in deep court, it doesn't mean that you should not attempt an offensive shot, only that your opponent has more time to react, has nobody to maneuver around, and has a clear view of the shot. In this case it is important to be accurate on your first attempt, because you probably will not get another chance.

While in deep court, try to create a situation that will move your opponent out of center court and let you move in. Two shots that will accomplish this are the *ceiling ball* and the *pass shot.* (See diagrams on page 56.) The ceiling ball is a defensive shot that is designed to have an opponent returning your shot from deep court while you are in center court. The pass shot is more of an offensive shot, designed to win the rally or leave your opponent struggling in deep court. When using these shots to extricate yourself from deep court, you will be playing the kind of smart, high-percentage racquetball it takes to win at this game.

Various positions from which to play center court

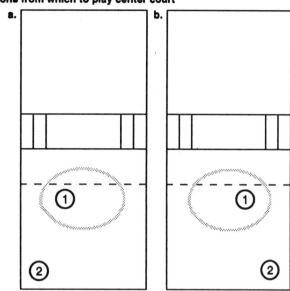

In (c), (d), and (e), player (1) can play from either position in center court.

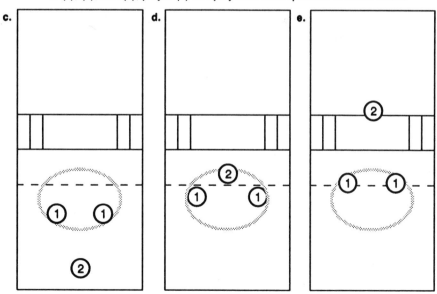

1 = player's position   2 = opponent's position

Flowing center court positions

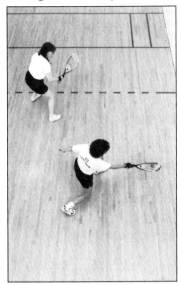

a.

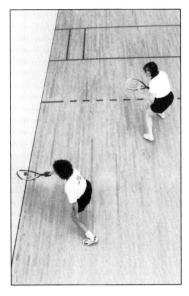

b.

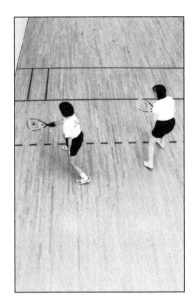

c.

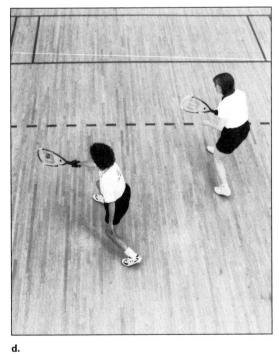

d.

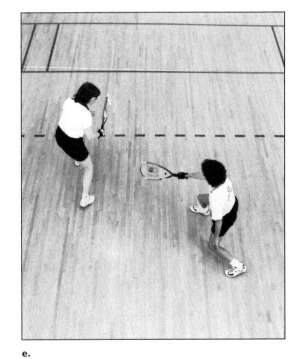

e.

Shots from deep court

a. Ceiling ball (2 shots):

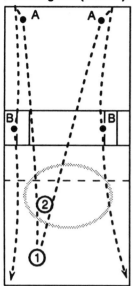

(A) ball hits ceiling,
(B) ball hits floor before
    bounce toward back
    wall.

b. Pass shot (2 shots)

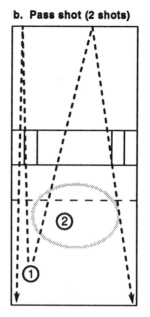

c. Side-by-side

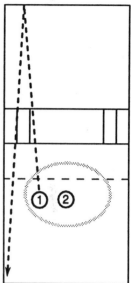

1 = player   2 = opponent

✓ *Checklist for Center Court Position*

1. Determine the lateral boundaries of your "flowing center court" by extending your arm until the racquet touches the side walls.
2. Take a position on the side of center court toward which your opponent is playing the shot.
3. Control center court by keeping your opponent in deep court.
4. When your opponent is controlling center court and you are stuck in deep court, use ceiling balls and pass shots to reverse the positions.

There are also situations that arise when neither person is in control of center court. One example is when both players are side by side. In this and similar situations, hit a shot that keeps your body between the opponent and the ball. This forces the opponent to take an indirect path around you to reach the ball, thus using up more time and energy.

Doubles Play

Doubles play is an exciting and enjoyable alternative to singles play. You will be challenged to use your entire shot selection, while moving out of the way of the ball and the other players, and to use your teamwork capabilities. With four people vying for the same territory, the court is crowded, but there actually is adequate room if you learn proper court positioning and the techniques of hitting and constantly moving.

The social aspect of doubles is an added attraction. You can enjoy playing racquetball with three friends and afterward discuss the game highlights and the friendly competition.

There are three basic styles of team doubles play:

- I-formation
- Side-by-side
- Staggered side-by-side

I-Formation

This style of play has one team member positioned in the middle of the front court and the second team member in the middle of the back court. The front player is responsible for any shot that stays in the front third of the court: all kill shots and pinch shots. This player should be the partner with the quicker reflexes, since the closer you play to the front wall the faster the ball returns. The backcourt player should be the one with the stronger stroke technique, since most returns will be made from deep in the court. This player is responsible for any shot that passes the player in front: all ceiling balls, pass shots, backwall shots.

Doubles positions
a. I-formation   **b. Side-by-side**   **c. and d. Staggered side-by-side**

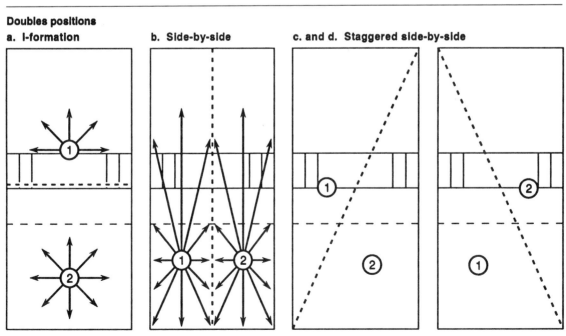

1 = first team   2 = second team

Doubles positions

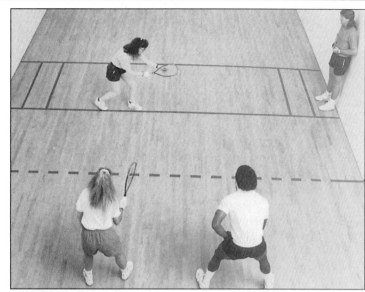

a. Serving

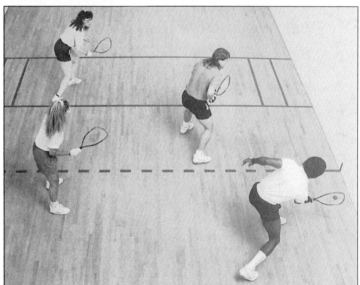

b. Server's partner moves into position after serve

Side-By-Side

Instead of dividing the court with a line from side wall to side wall (like the I-formation), this style divides the court with an imaginary line down the middle of the court, from front wall to back wall. Each player has total responsibility for the half of the court he or she is assigned; right or left. Shots hit to the middle of the court are played by the player on the left side of the court; the one with the forehand shot (assuming both players are right handed). If one partner is right-handed and the other left-handed, the left-handed player should play on the left side. This means that shots hit into either corner will be returned by a forehand.

Staggered Side-By-Side

This style of doubles team play is the most popular and probably the most effective method of covering the court. Each player adjusts his or her coverage according to the position of the ball on the court. If your partner moves forward, you move back; if you move forward, your partner moves back.

When you are the player positioned in the front, you cover the front wall for kill shots and pinch shots, and any down-the-wall pass shots that are hit along the wall on your side of the court. If you are the player positioned in the rear, you are responsible for any shots that pass your partner, travel along the wall on your side of the court, or end up in deep court. Even though the partners adjust their position according to where the ball is, it is good strategy to have the quicker player in the front as often as possible. Fast hands and quick feet are an important asset when playing close to the front wall.

Serving in Doubles

Right Side Player

As the right side player, you will have the difficult task of usually serving to your opponent's forehand. Don't let this intimidate you. Remember that you have two people covering the return. Even though it will usually be a forehand return, it places twice as much pressure on the receiver to make a perfect shot.

A drive serve down the wall can be an effective serve, providing it does not rebound from the back wall or contact the side wall and rebound toward the center. This leaves the receiver a clear, wide lane along the wall in which to play the shot.

Z serves are an excellent choice because they enable your partner to move up to cover the short game, while you can cover shots down the line.

High lobs to the opponent's forehand often force forehand ceiling ball returns, which allow you and your partner adequate time to get out of the service zone and into good playing position. This may cause problems for some players who do not practice these returns.

A jam serve takes a path toward both players. It pressures your opponents into making a quick decision as to which one will return the serve.

Left Side Player

All of the same serves apply to the left side player as to the right side player. When on the left side, you will be serving mostly to your opponent's backhand, but don't be afraid to serve straight down the middle of the court to keep the receiver off balance. You also may want to hit serves that use the near, side wall to create different angles and looks to your serve.

Playing a "Lefty/Righty" Team

Usually, the strongest doubles teams consist of a left-handed player and a right-handed player. With the left-handed player playing on the left side and right-handed player on the right side, this team has a distinct advantage because both players can hit forehand shots on balls hit to either side of the court. It is very difficult to serve effectively to this type of team because most players are accustomed to serving a large majority of their serves toward their opponents' backhand. This is also true during rallies. When a player hits a ball into either corner, instead of the usual backhand return, the result is always a forehand.

To be successful against this combination, place your shots into the middle of the court, where either opponent is forced to use a backhand return and to quickly decide which one will hit the return. Jam serves are an excellent choice for this purpose. Using the same strategy, hit ceiling balls away from the corners and more toward the center of the court. Before you walk on the court, discuss with your partner this particular game plan that can be employed against this lefty/righty combination.

 ## Checklist for Rules of Doubles Play

While you can choose from several game plans for doubles play, there are some basic rules that you should apply to your strategy.

1. Do *not* yell at your partner or make faces when he misses a shot. Doubles is a *team game*. Partners need to communicate in order to work together as a smooth unit. It is important to encourage and support your partner, not ridicule or undermine him or her. It helps to realize that when you have to "carry" a partner who plays poorly one day, there may be another day when the roles are reversed. *Be good to your partner!*

2. Do *not* serve behind your partner (to your partner's side of the court) without a signal. When you serve to your partner's side of the court, you put him or her in a dangerous situation. Your partner is confined to the doubles service box and is stranded along the wall and vulnerable to the danger of being hit by a very hard shot. If you do decide to serve behind your partner, devise a signal to enable him or her to move out of the box quickly and be ready for the return. *Be good to your partner!*

3. If your partner dives or falls and is lying on the floor, or is stranded in front court, make your next shot a ceiling ball. You can't play doubles alone, so allow time for your partner to get up, return to a better position, and get out of danger. Even if you have a set-up to score a point, pass it up in order to protect your partner. *Be good to your partner!*

4. Play your own shots in your own designated side or area. This rule applies to all levels of doubles play, but especially to mixed doubles play (a team of one male and one female). Do not hog your partner's shots or force him or her into the back corner so you can play a singles match. Doubles is a team game; two people, playing their own shots in their own area. *Be good to your partner!*

Checklist for Doubles Tips

1. Take a position away from the side wall. Once you get trapped against the wall, there is no room to move or swing. *Stay away from the wall!*

2. Watch the ball at all times. Since there are four players on the court it is crucial that you know where everyone is positioned so you can stay out of the way. If you plant yourself and stare at the front wall waiting for the ball to rebound, you will be in someone's way. It is your responsibility to move out of the way of an opponent's shot to avoid causing a hinder.

3. Communicate with your partner. Get in the habit of talking during rallies. It is fine to yell out "mine" or "yours" so there is no doubt about who will take the shot.

4. Safety first! Be aware of the other players on the court and hold up your shot if necessary. It is better to play a rally over than to accidentally hit someone with the ball or your racquet.

5. Have fun. Doubles is a great game!

Summary

1. Always be ready to move by staying in the ready position.
2. Unless you have to race to a distant part of the court, shuffle to the ball with a step-together-step movement.
3. Concentrating on the ball will help you to anticipate your opponent's next shot.
4. Controlling "flowing center court" offers many advantages, such as the following:
   - The opportunity to attack with offensive shots
   - Being in position to reach more of your opponent's shots
   - Your opponent will be forced to retrieve your shot from deep court
   - Your opponent will be forced to run around you
   - Your body might block your opponent's view of the ball
5. When your opponent is in control of center court, use ceiling balls or pass shots to force him or her into deep court and allow you to recapture center court.
6. Doubles play can be a challenge to your shot selection, mobility, and teamwork skills. It also adds a dimension of sociability to the game.
7. There are three basic styles of doubles court coverage: I-formation, side-by-side, and staggered side-by-side.
8. Serving in doubles can create different problems: receivers are positioned in either corner, your partner is in a position that forces you to constantly serve to a forehand, and righty/lefty combinations that challenge you to play down the middle to avoid forehand returns. Proper serve selection can help to alleviate these problems.
9. Be good to your partner! Doubles is a team game.

Defensive Shots

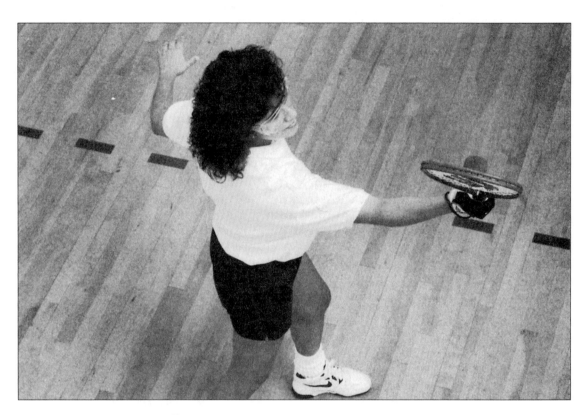

Outline

Defensive shots are a variety of plays that are made with the objective of keeping your opponent from having a good scoring opportunity and increasing your chances of getting another shot before the end of the rally. Ceiling balls (shots), around-the-wall balls, and "Z" balls are all designed to get players out of trouble and keep them in the rally. Since players generally do not plan to score from these shots, they are called *defensive shots.* Actually, every shot does have the potential to score, and if a player stays alert, these three shots can be aggressive and intelligent shots to utilize in that way.

An example of aggressively using a defensive shot is hitting a ceiling ball after you have hit a series of kill shots. As your opponent charges to front court to intercept the expected kill shot, the ball bounces high into deep court, forcing your opponent to stop short, change direction, reverse his or her forward momentum, and hurry to the rear wall to return the shot. It is not so important whether or not the opponent makes this shot, because this action will affect future kill shot situations—the chance of another ceiling shot will cause your opponent to hesitate, allowing you more leeway on kill shots.

Another bonus of using defensive shots is that you are getting into your opponent's head, using psychological warfare to make the opponent worry about shot selection. Even though it is done with defense in mind—keeping your opponent from getting a good scoring opportunity and providing a chance to prolong the rally—this type of play can work offensively as well.

Ceiling Ball

A consistent, accurate *ceiling ball* is a necessary and important weapon in the arsenal of an all-around player. A ceiling ball can give you time to recover the mid-court area when you're out of position by forcing your opponent back and away from the mid-court area.

Weapon and *arsenal* are aggressive words, used purposely to avoid having the reader think, "Ho-hum, here comes the boring ceiling shot section." It is impossible to win at "shoot-out" racquetball without something to back up the artillery of offensive attack strategies. A solid ceiling game is that all-important element.

Target Point

The ceiling ball should be aimed to hit the ceiling before making contact with the front wall. Using this shot will cause the ball to land on the floor in the vicinity of the service zone and then bounce high into deep court, forcing your opponent to move back near the rear wall.

The closer to the ceiling crotch (the corner between the ceiling and front wall) the ball hits, the deeper it will land. The farther back on the ceiling (away from the crotch) the ball hits, the farther from the back wall the ball will bounce.

Each player needs to learn to make adjustments as to which point on the ceiling to direct the ball toward, as this depends on the speed of the ball, the

Path of ceiling shot

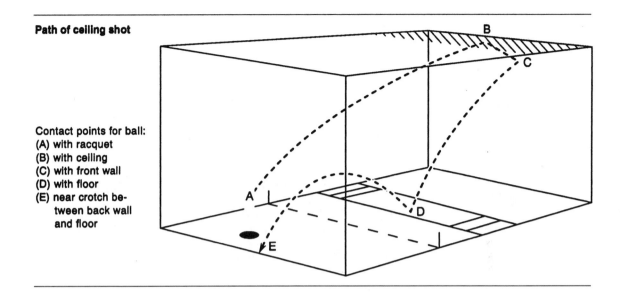

Contact points for ball:
(A) with racquet
(B) with ceiling
(C) with front wall
(D) with floor
(E) near crotch be-
     tween back wall
     and floor

strength of the stroke, and the height at the point of contact.

When a lively ball causes your ceiling shots to rebound from the back wall and sets up your opponent with kill shots, instead of softer shots, make your shot contact with the ceiling farther back from the front wall. This will cause the ball to land before it hits the back wall.

For all ceiling shots, the racquet face should go from a low position to a high position; "low to high, low to high" is a catchphrase to help you concentrate on ceiling shots.

Forehand Ceiling Ball

The motion for the *forehand ceiling ball* is similar to that of throwing a baseball over a high wall. Your body should be turned facing the side wall, as in all other shots. For the overhead ceiling ball, bring the racquet back behind your head and, using an easy motion, swing up through the ball, letting the follow-through finish near the opposite thigh. Step into the shot, just as with all of the other shots discussed earlier, and swing up with an easy motion. This shot does not have to be blasted.

Backhand Ceiling Ball

The *backhand ceiling ball* is hit with the same basic technique as the backhand stroke, except that the swing is up, through the ball, toward the ceiling. Your body is turned toward the side wall and your shoulders should be pulled all the way back. Step diagonally toward the ball and make contact even with your front foot, at face or head level. Follow through until your arm is fully extended and the racquet is pointing toward the ceiling.

Forehand ceiling shot ball: from behind and from above

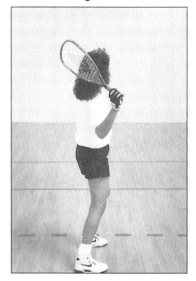

a. Backswing

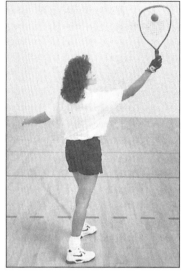

b. Swing and contact

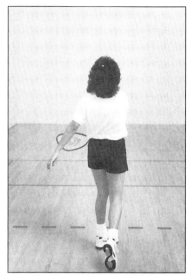

c. Follow-through

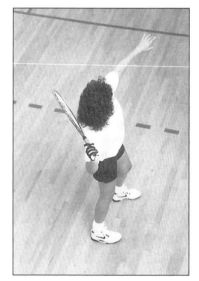

d. Backswing

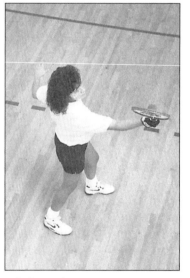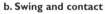

e. Swing and contact

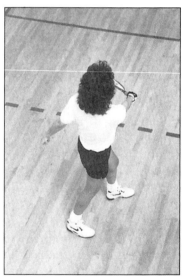

f. Follow-through

For all ceiling shots, whether underhand or overhand, the racquet will go from low to high. Aim the racquet at the ceiling first, not at a side wall or the front wall. By hitting the ceiling first, the ball should bounce to the front wall, then down near the service court, then deep into the back court where it should land without hitting the back wall. This forces your opponent back and out of the offensive part of the court.

Backhand ceiling ball: from behind and from above

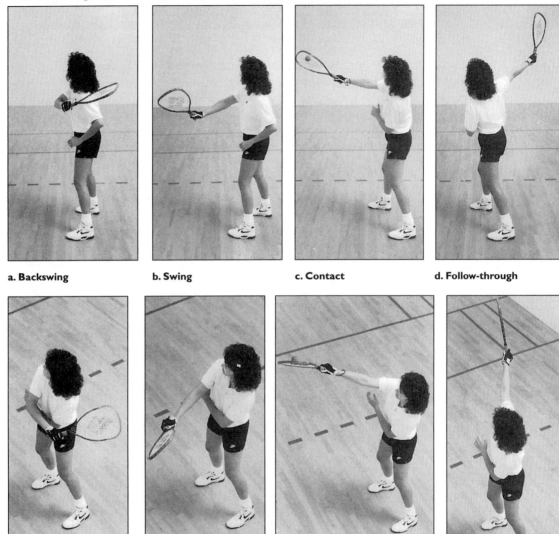

| a. Backswing | b. Swing | c. Contact | d. Follow-through |

| e. Backswing | f. Swing | g. Contact | h. Follow-through |

Use of Ceiling Balls

When to use a ceiling ball:

1. After an opponent has hit a ceiling ball that bounds above your head. Instead of attempting a lower-percentage offensive shot, like an overhead smash or passing shot, hit a return ceiling shot and wait for a better set up.

Checklist for Ceiling Balls

1. The target point should be on the ceiling, close to the front wall.
2. Properly executed ceiling shots will force an opponent into deep court.
3. Ceiling shots should bounce a second time before making contact with the back wall.
4. Learn to make adjustments related to the speed of the ball and the power of your shot.
5. The closer to the front wall you hit the ball, the deeper it will land in the court.
6. The racquet face should go from a low position to a high position; remember the phrase "low to high."
7. The motion for a forehand ceiling shot is similar to that of throwing a baseball over a high wall.
8. The backhand ceiling shot is hit up, through the ball, toward the ceiling.
9. The shot should be directed at the ceiling, not at a side wall.

2. **As a service return.** A ceiling ball is always a wise choice, especially at the beginning and intermediate levels. It starts a rally, forces the server out of center court, and allows the receiver to take over the offensive, center court position.

3. **When you're out of position or hitting off balance.** Hitting a ceiling ball will buy you precious time to recover and get back into the rally.

4. **When you're tired or winded.** Hitting a series of ceiling balls can give you some time to recover and regain strength, because this shot is made with an easier stroke and, in effect, slows the pace of the game while the players exchange ceiling balls.

5. **When playing an opponent who likes to play a hard and fast style of game.** Use ceiling balls to take this type of opponent out of his or her desired game plan.

6. **When playing against a player who has a great kill shot.** Using a ceiling shot will minimize that player's chances of getting into the scoring zone.

Around-the-Wall Ball

The *around-the-wall ball* is a change of pace from the ceiling ball. While it also ends up in deep court, it takes a different, roundabout path to get there.

Begin the shot from a position near one of the side walls and aim for a spot about 15 feet high on the opposite side wall, about five to six feet back from the front wall. The ball will quickly make contact with the front wall, bouncing well behind the service line, before hitting the other side wall in deep court. The shot may be executed with either a forehand or backhand stroke. The hitting motion is similar to the ceiling ball, except that the racquet face is angled

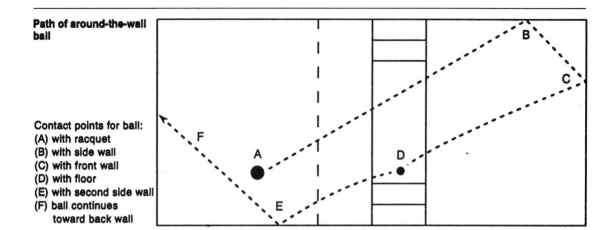

Path of around-the-wall ball

Contact points for ball:
(A) with racquet
(B) with side wall
(C) with front wall
(D) with floor
(E) with second side wall
(F) ball continues
    toward back wall

high on the side wall, not toward the ceiling. (This shot can be very confusing to beginning-level players because of the angles, changes in direction, and the different spin put on the ball as it comes off of the walls.)

When playing this shot, there is no need to go chasing all over the court. Wait patiently for the ball in the middle of the deep back court and it will come to you. Then hit a ceiling ball or another around-the-wall shot and continue the rally.

One danger of this shot is that the ball travels through the center court area, allowing an alert opponent to cut it off in the air, thus leaving the shooter stranded in deep court. Around-the-wall shots can be made more effective when hit at varying speeds and heights; hit high and soft one time and the next time hit low and with more power, whipping the ball around the walls. Changing height and velocity makes it difficult for an opponent to anticipate when to cut the shot off.

Use of the Around-the-Wall Ball

When to use the around-the-wall ball:
1. During a rally, after a number of ceiling balls have been hit. The spin and change of directions may disrupt an opponent's timing and cause him or her to make a poor shot.
2. Against a player who is not accustomed to the shot. Try it a few times early in a game and see how your opponent reacts; then use the shot accordingly.
3. As a change of pace.

The "Z" Ball

The *"Z" ball* is an often-overlooked defensive shot that can add flair and distinction to one's game. It is a wild-looking shot that gets its name for the "Z" pattern it makes as it hits the walls. It is the most offensive of the defensive shots and may even score a point.

Checklist for the Around-the-Wall Ball

1. Begin the shot from a position near one of the side walls.
2. The ball should first make contact with the opposite side wall about five feet from the front wall and about fifteen feet high.
3. The stroke is similar to that used with the ceiling ball, except that the racquet is angled at the side wall.
4. One danger of this shot is that it crosses center court and may be cut off by an alert opponent.
5. Change height and velocity to keep an opponent off balance.

This shot should always be hit into the opposite corner from a position near one of the side walls, and it may be executed either forehand or backhand. It is hit like an around-the-wall shot, except it makes contact with the front wall first. After hitting the front wall, about twelve to sixteen feet high and two or three feet from the side wall, it then hits one side wall and rebounds directly to the opposite side wall, after which it bounces nearly parallel to and about two or three feet from the back wall. This angle makes it a difficult shot to return, because there is very little room to get behind the ball and hit it toward the front wall.

The "Z" ball should be attempted only when you are within its target range—the area in the vicinity of the service zone and no more than about five feet behind the service line. If hit from the wrong area of the court, the desired angles cannot be achieved.

The reason many players enjoy using this shot is because it can potentially embarrass an opponent, which may be good for an extra point or two during the game. When an alert opponent moves forward to cover the low shot expected from a front court set up, flick your wrist at the last second and send the ball toward the top of the corner. This will cause your opponent to stop short, reverse his or her momentum, and head for deep court, only to find that the ball is going in a different direction. This makes the opponent feel self-conscious and frustrated. Not only can you score a point, but using this tactic can have a negative psychological effect on your opponent.

Use of the "Z" Ball

When to use the "Z" ball:

1. When in trouble due to being off balance or out of position.
2. Occasionally, to keep your opponent off balance and unsure of whether to hang back or charge when mid-court set ups occur.
3. Only when you are within the suggested range or can achieve the appropriate angle, because otherwise you'll be giving your opponent an easy shot off of the back wall.

Path of z-ball

Contact points for ball:
(A) with racquet
(B) with front wall
(C) with side wall
(D) with second side wall
(E) ball rebounds
    parallel to back wall

Target zones for around-the-wall ball and z-ball

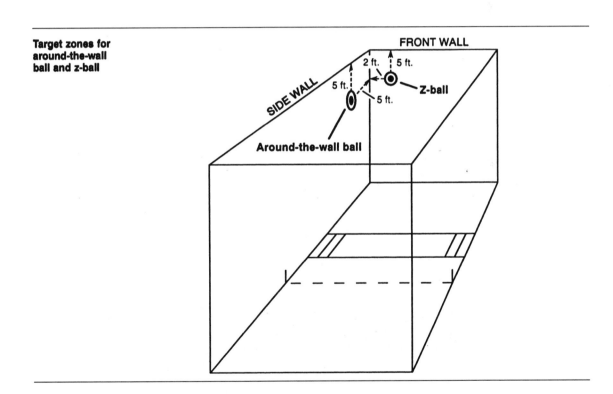

Checklist for the "Z" Ball

1. Hit the "Z" ball from a position near one of the side walls.
2. The "Z" ball hits the front wall first, twelve to sixteen feet high and two or three feet from the side wall.
3. Attempt this shot only in the vicinity of the service zone.
4. Use this shot as a change of pace to confuse an opponent.

Back Wall to Front Wall Shot

The *back wall to front wall shot* should be used only as a last resort, when there is no way to make the ball go directly toward the front wall or when it is the only remaining way to keep the ball in play.

This shot is hit directly into the back wall and must hit the front wall before it hits the floor. When you're not in position to return the ball toward the front wall, hit the ball hard, directly into the back wall, at an angle that will allow the ball to hit near the front-wall ceiling crotch. This will result in a high bounce and force the opponent to play the shot in the back court. The shot can be executed with either a forehand or backhand stroke, and is more effective if kept close to one of the side walls.

The angle must be such that the ball, after making contact with the back wall, hits the front wall near the ceiling. If the angle is too low, it will usually result in an easy set up for your opponent, with you stuck in the deep court. The stroke is similar to a ceiling ball, except that if it is hit at too high an angle, it will not reach the front wall. And note that even if it's hit correctly, this shot may be cut off on the fly or short-hop by an aggressive opponent.

Players who rely on this shot develop lazy habits—they hang back in the deep court and become less aggressive. Many beginners use this shot to avoid hitting shots off of the back wall. This inhibits them from developing the back-wall skills necessary to become a complete player.

 Checklist for Back Wall to Front Wall Shot

1. Use only when there is no other way to get the ball to the front wall.
2. The ball is hit directly into the back wall, with enough velocity so it will hit the front wall before making contact with the floor.
3. The ball must be hit hard, with a stroke similar to that used for a ceiling ball.
4. The ball must be hit at an angle that will enable it to hit near the front-wall ceiling crotch.
5. Try to keep this shot as close to a side wall as possible.
6. This shot can be used from a forehand or backhand stroke.

Path of backwall to frontwall shot

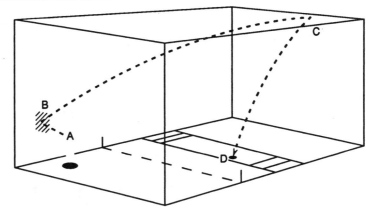

Contact points for ball:
(A) with racquet
(B) with back wall
(C) near front wall/
**   ceiling crotch**
(D) with floor

✓	*Checklist for Defensive Shots*

1. The ceiling ball, around-the-wall ball, and "Z" ball are the primary defensive shots.
2. Defensive shots drive the opponent from center court to a deep court position.
3. Use defensive shots as a change of pace from the shoot-out-style of play.
4. Be prepared to make individual adjustments, depending on the liveliness of the ball and your power level.
5. Balls aimed near the front-wall ceiling crotch must be hit from low to high.
6. Use defensive shots when an opponent has an advantage or when a high-percentage offensive shot is not available.
7. Use defensive shots when a rest is needed.
8. Changing velocity on defensive shots can confuse and keep an opponent off balance.
9. Defensive shots are necessary to an all-around game.

Summary

1. The objective of a defensive shot is to keep an opponent from getting a set up and extending the rally.
2. All shots have the potential to score.
3. Defensive shots can give the player a psychological advantage, by upsetting the opponent's game plan and turning him or her off balance.
4. Ceiling balls, around-the-wall balls, "Z" balls, and back wall to front wall shots are considered defensive shots.
5. Ceiling balls are hit from low to high.
6. Back wall to front wall shots should be used only as a last resort.
7. Defensive shots should be used when a high-percentage shot is not available or when the opponent has a better court position.

7 *Offensive Shots*

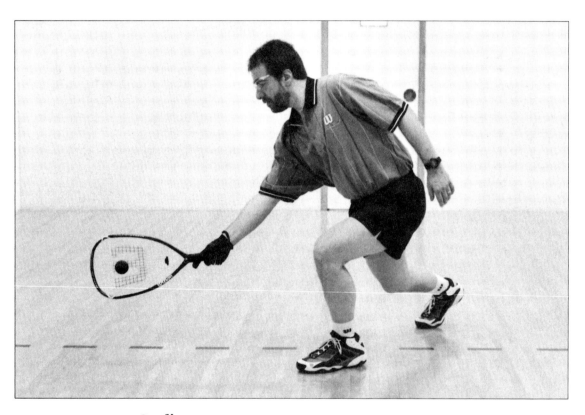

Outline

I n order to win consistently in racquetball, it is essential to possess the skills to hit offensive shots. Offensive shots end rallies and score points. Defensive shots extend rallies and help players recover from difficult situations. The difference between offensive and defensive shots are that offensive shots mean playing to win, while defensive shots mean playing to not lose.

This chapter will discuss the ultimate offensive shots; why, how, and when to use them as the key to a power game.

The Kill Shot

The *kill shot* is the Rolls Royce of offensive shots. There is no defense against a properly executed kill shot. A kill shot will end a rally immediately and definitely. In order to play an aggressive, winning style of racquetball, a kill shot must be a part of a player's arsenal.

A kill shot is any shot hit low enough on the front wall so that it will take two quick bounces before an opponent can reach it. The second bounce usually occurs before the ball reaches the service zone.

A spectacular variation of a kill shot is a *roll out,* a ball that hits so low on the front wall that it rolls back along the floor without any bounce. Needless to say, this is a very rare shot.

In order for a kill shot to be effective, it must hit low enough on the front wall that it will not rebound to the mid-court area. In order to keep the ball down, contact with the ball must be made low.

The contact area for both forehand and backhand strokes is anywhere between mid-thigh to mid-calf, depending on the type of shot selected. When a decision is made to hit a kill shot, the point of contact should be in the mid-calf range. This means letting the ball drop until it is at the desired height. It takes discipline and patience to avoid rushing and making contact with the ball before it drops to this lower contact point.

You may have to make adjustments to the point of contact, depending on the area of the court from which the shot is attempted; hit it a little higher if you are positioned deeper, and a little lower if you are in the front court. Generally, though, mid-calf is the contact point for kill shots.

All racquetball shots can be difficult to learn and require many hours of practice, but the kill shot is especially difficult. Since the target is the bottom few inches on the front wall, it leaves little room for error. The chances of committing an error can be minimized by knowing your scoring zone.

Scoring Zone

Scoring zones are the areas in which a player can consistently be successful with a shot. If a player's kill shot is accurate from twenty feet or closer, that would be his or her scoring zone. For this player, it would not be a good shot selection to attempt a kill shot at game point from thirty-six feet.

As a player's skill level increases, the scoring zone will broaden, increasing the opportunities and areas from which one may safely attempt kill shots.

The whole purpose of hitting a kill shot is to end rallies and score points. Since it is so difficult to defend, a barrage of kill shots can quickly demoralize

Path of straight kill shot

A
B
D
C

Contact points for ball:
(A) with racquet
(B) with front wall
(C) with floor:
    first bounce
(D) with floor:
    second bounce

an opponent. The main question is when to hit a kill shot. The more experienced a player is, the easier it is to recognize kill shot opportunities. A kill shot is exciting and well-worth the practice time it takes to develop consistency and confidence in making it.

Use of the Kill Shot

When to use the kill shot:

1. When you're in center court and your opponent is behind you. Even if the shot hits too high on the wall, the opponent will have to run a long way to get to the ball.

2. When a ball rebounds from the back wall toward the mid-court area and into your scoring zone.

3. When a ball drops into your scoring zone, either from a short ceiling ball or directly from a side wall. (Be aggressive and try to end the rally.)

4. When there is adequate time to set up. If the ball is in your scoring zone, plant your feet and attack.

✓ Checklist for the Kill Shot

1. The contact point for the kill shot is at mid-calf level.
2. At the point of contact, the racquet strings face the front wall.
3. To make a level swing, wait until the ball drops to the desired level. A level swing will make the ball hit low on the front wall.
4. The target point is the bottom few inches on the front wall.
5. A kill shot should bounce twice before reaching mid-court.
6. Adjust the contact height to the situation: higher when hitting from back court and lower when hitting from front court.
7. Recognize kill shot opportunities within your own scoring zone.

Contact for kill shots

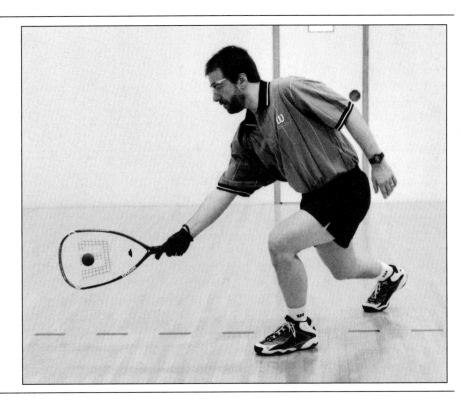

The Pinch Shot

If the kill shot is the Rolls Royce of offensive shots, the *pinch shot* is the Lamborghini. It is a very effective, exotic-looking shot, and one that is not used often enough.

The pinch shot is a variation of the kill shot. The difference is that it hits two walls instead of one. The ball hits low and tight into the side wall/front wall corner, making a little "boom-boom" sound as it hits both walls in rapid succession. It should hit the side wall first. A pinch shot is hit the same way as a kill shot, by letting the ball drop to mid-calf level and swinging through it. The difference is that with the pinch shot, the ball is aimed at a side wall instead of straight at the front wall. This difference begins with the angle of the racquet strings.

For a straight kill shot, the racquet strings are facing the front wall when the arm is fully extended. With a pinch shot the strings face towards a side wall instead of the front wall. This is accomplished by slightly bending your wrist back, allowing the strings to angle toward a side wall. The ball goes wherever the strings face.

Envision a pool table. Now, think of a racquetball court as a big pool table. A pinch shot should put the ball in the side pockets. Where the ball hits dictates where you put the ball on the side wall to create the correct angle to put the ball in the "side pocket."

A general rule of thumb is that the closer the ball is to the side wall, the deeper, or farther back on the side wall, you hit. As the ball moves farther away from the side wall, the farther up you hit.

Pool Table Diagram

Pinch Shots

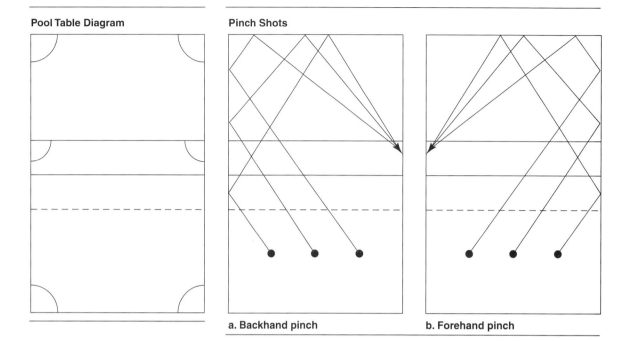

a. Backhand pinch   b. Forehand pinch

Beginning players often wonder why they should bother with a pinch shot if a kill shot is more effective. The reason is that the pinch shot is the only one that will force an opponent to run forward into the front court. The shot hits into the corner and, as it rebounds, the ball angles across the court instead of heading straight toward the back wall.

The result of this angle is that your opponent has to run forward to try to retrieve the shot. It is good strategy to force an opponent to travel over as much territory as possible; this is especially effective when both players are in the back court. Kill shots and pass shots move opponents from side to side, ceiling balls move them back, and pinch shots move them forward.

The pinch shot is a necessary weapon for an all-around game. Even though a missed pinch shot may leave the ball up in center court—a set up for your opponent—it is well worth the risk.

Another offensive technique is a *drop,* or *touch shot,* which is often used by finesse players to take advantage of a slow opponent; one who anticipates a ceiling ball, pass shot, or other hard shot; or one who remains in deep court. This type of shot is most effective when hit as a pinch shot, a surprise, or a change of pace. The shot involves learning to hit the ball softly, with a pushing motion. Each individual will need to experiment to find the right touch. The danger of this shot is that the ball could remain suspended, giving your opponent a "plum" set up.

Use of the Pinch Shot

When to use the pinch shot:

1. When you want a slow opponent to travel as great a distance as possible.

Wrist action

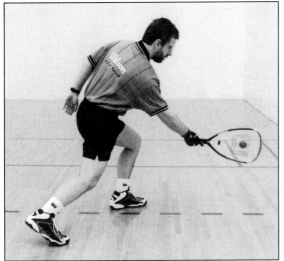

a. Kill shot

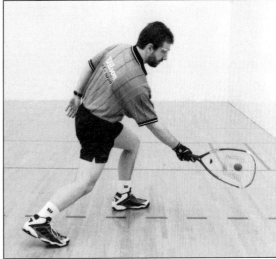

b. Pinch shot

   Checklist for the Pinch Shot

1. The pinch shot is a kill shot hit into either front corner.
2. At the point of contact, the racquet strings face a side wall.
3. Pinch shots will force an opponent to move forward.
4. Pinch shots can be used in any situation that calls for a kill shot.
5. Use pinch shots when both players are in the backcourt.

2. When both players are in deep court (assuming you are in your scoring zone).
3. When your opponent is stranded near a side wall. A pinch shot to that side will make the ball rebound toward the opposite wall.
4. Any situation that calls for a kill shot. A pinch shot is a kill shot that hits two walls.
5. When an opponent is behind you.

The Pass Shot

The *pass shot* is any ball that goes past an opponent and ends up in the back part of the court. It should be hit just low enough so that it won't reach the back wall before it bounces twice; this way, your opponent won't get a second chance. A pass shot should be hit to an area of the court where your opponent is not positioned.

Pass shot contact and wrist action

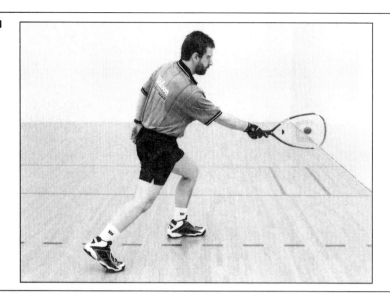

Pass shots

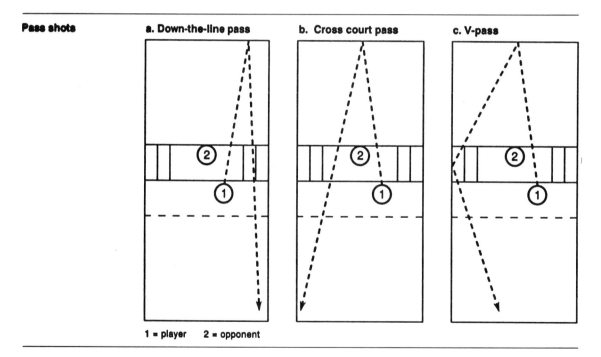

a. Down-the-line pass   b. Cross court pass   c. V-pass

1 = player   2 = opponent

Pass shots are an important way to balance kill shot attempts. Diversity is a must in order to keep an opponent off balance. A successful pass shot will force an opponent into deep back court and allow you to move into the strategic center court position.

The pass shot should be hit higher on the front wall than a kill shot or pinch shot, and your point of contact with the ball is also higher—somewhere between the knee and mid-thigh. A level swing will make the ball hit higher on the front wall and then drive past your opponent.

There are three basic types of pass shots:
- Down the line
- Cross court
- "V"

Down-the-Line Pass

The *down-the-line pass* is hit parallel, near the wall on the shooter's side of the court. (For a right-hander, it is the right side for a forehand and the left side for a backhand.) It is a difficult shot to hit effectively, but a very handy weapon to develop. Generally, when you hit a forehand, your opponent will be closer than you to the center of the court. A down-the-line shot will force your opponent to move farther away from the center of the court.

One of the keys to this shot is to keep the racquet face parallel to the front wall, or the shot will angle toward the side wall. If this happens, the ball will end up in center court instead of continuing along the side wall.

Cross-Court Pass

The *cross-court pass* does what it says it will do—travel from one side of the court to the other—at about a forty-five degree angle to the opposite rear corner. The target area is very close to the center of the front wall. This pass shot will prevent an opponent from leaning (or "cheating") toward one side of the court. It also causes an opponent to make a full pivot and move in the opposite direction from where he or she was originally facing.

It is an easier shot to accomplish than a down-the-wall pass, because of the larger target area—the entire front wall—which leaves more margin for error.

"V" Pass or Wide Angle Pass

A *"V" pass* is a finesse shot that is seldom used, even on the professional level. It is a cross-court pass that hits the front wall with a wide angle, close to the opposite corner. The shot is intended to then hit the side wall at about the same depth as your opponent is positioned, bouncing behind the opponent. The "V" refers to the path of the ball after it rebounds from the side wall.

If hit well, this shot is virtually unretrievable. Unlike the other pass shots, even if the "V" shot is hit too high, it is still more difficult to play because of the angle of the ball and the spin it creates. While the down-the-line and cross-court pass shots can be hit from nearly anywhere on the court, the "V" pass is limited to a certain target zone, one that will provide the correct angle. This is an advanced shot and should be added to a player's repertoire only after he or she has mastered the down-the-line and cross-court passes. (If you hit one accidentally and are successful, smile and pretend you did it on purpose)

Checklist for the Pass Shot

1. A pass shot should be hit just hard enough to bounce twice before reaching the back wall.
2. Use pass shots to move an opponent to a rear corner.
3. Pass shots hit higher on the front wall than kill shots, as the result of a level swing at mid-thigh level.
4. Use pass shots to move an opponent away from center court position, or if the opponent is out of position.
5. The down-the-line pass is hit parallel and near a side wall. Be sure to keep the racquet strings parallel to the front wall at contact, or the ball will strike the side wall and rebound into center court.
6. The target area for the cross-court pass is near the center of the front wall, ending up in the opposite rear corner.
7. The target area for a "V" pass on the front wall is closer to the opposite wall, and should then hit the side wall even with the opponent's position.

Use of the Pass Shot

When to use the pass shot:

1. When the opponent has a good position in center court and you are in deep court. A pass shot will force the opponent to run after the shot, giving up center court position.
2. When the opponent is squared off and facing the front wall. It is difficult to pivot quickly from this position.
3. When both players are in the center court area. The opponent may be leaning forward, expecting a kill shot. The passing shot will keep him or her off balance and unsure of what strategy you will use.
4. When opponent is out of position in mid-court or front court.

The Overhead Shot

The *overhead shot* has gained in popularity over the last few years, especially at the higher levels of play. The shot was originally used mainly by converted tennis players who had already developed this technique from service play. The racquetball population finally decided to adopt it, and now it is a common shot.

The overhead shot is a lower-percentage shot in terms of overall consistency, which is the reason it is used mainly by higher-skilled players. But it is a shot that is a lot of fun to hit, and it can give added dimension to an attack style of play.

There are two types of overheads: the *drive* and the *kill.* Both are hit with the same motion; the difference is the angle of the racquet face.

The motion of the overhead stroke is similar to the ceiling ball (see Chapter 6) except that instead of aiming the racquet face at the ceiling, the wrist swings over the top until the racquet strings are facing the lower part of the front wall. The motion is similar to a tennis serve or to throwing a baseball toward the ground about 10 feet in front of you.

Overhead Drive

The *overhead drive* is usually hit from deep court when playing a ceiling ball that is dropping before hitting the back wall. In order to attempt this shot, the ball should be higher than your head (hence the name *overhead*). The target point on the front wall is three to four feet above the floor so that it rebounds past the opponent, either down the line or cross court. The result of this shot is that your opponent moves out of center court.

Another technique is to make the ball rebound directly at the opponent's body, forcing him or her into making a reaction shot, hopefully resulting in a set up for you.

To be successful, this shot must be kept from rebounding from the back wall, which will set your opponent up for a kill shot. This can be accomplished by hitting the ball lower on the front wall or by hitting it with a softer touch, slowing the pace or velocity of the shot.

Use of the Overhead Drive

When to use the overhead drive:
1. When a change of pace is needed in a ceiling-ball rally.
2. When the opponent is content to play a safe, slow game.
3. When your game plan is to constantly attack throughout the game.

Overhead Kill Shot

This is an extremely difficult shot to master and is not worth a lot of practice. Unless the *overhead kill* is hit perfectly, it will skip on the floor or end up in front court, giving your opponent an easy set up. It is a very low-percentage shot and more often results in failure than with a kill.

In spite of its drawbacks, a number of players do decide to attempt the overhead kill. The motion is the same as for an overhead drive shot, except the target area is as low as possible in either front corner, ending with a pinch shot.

The only feasible opportunity to attempt this shot is when an opponent is in deep court, anticipating a ceiling ball. When executing the shot, wait until the last second to snap your wrist down and over the ball, in the hope that your opponent will be caught flat-footed, which allows you some margin of error in your placement of the shot.

Overhead shot: from front and above

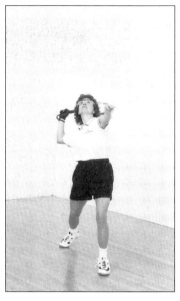

a. Backswing

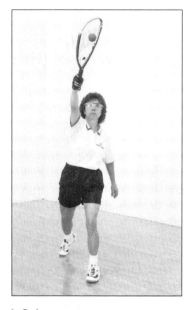

b. Swing

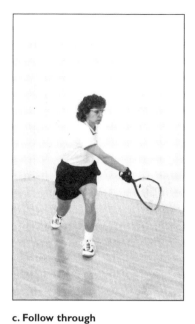

c. Follow through

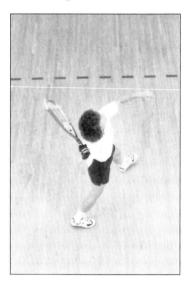

d. Backswing

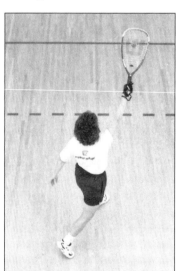

e. Swing and contact

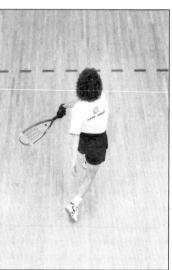

f. Follow through

Use of the Overhead Kill Shot

When to use the overhead kill shot:

1. Very rarely, since it is a very low-percentage shot.

2. When your opponent is in deep court, anticipating a ceiling ball, or when he or she is flat-footed or just lazy.

3. As a surprise shot, to throw a monkey wrench into your opponent's game plan.

Checklist for the Overhead Shot

1. The overhead stroke is similar to a tennis serve or throwing a baseball at the ground.
2. The wrist swings over the top until the racquet face is aimed at the lower part of the front wall.
3. The overhead drive, hit from deep court, should rebound past the opponent down the line, cross court, or directly at an opponent.
4. The overhead drive should be kept from rebounding off the back wall.
5. On an overhead kill shot, the target is lower on the front wall, and is more effective as a pinch shot.
6. Use the overhead kill only when an opponent is in deep court, expecting a ceiling ball.

The Jam Shot

The *jam shot* is a very enjoyable, off-beat type of shot that can give an opponent fits, and it can be an effective shot at any skill level. What makes this shot so much fun is that opponents do not believe that you did it on purpose. This frustrates them, because they think the rally was won by a lucky or fluke shot.

Most shots are designed to fly away from opponents, forcing them to run and hit the ball while on the move. A jam shot works on the opposite theory—hit the ball so that it rebounds up, into the opponent's body, "handcuffing" the opponent so he can't make a shot or forcing a reaction shot or an attempt to just block the ball's path.

The jam shot is hit like a pass shot, except the target zone is on the front wall directly in front of your opponent, making the ball rebound straight into the opponent's body. It is most effective when hit with full power, but if this is not possible due to lack of time or poor position, aim for a spot a little higher on the wall so the ball gets to your opponent more quickly.

Checklist for the Jam Shot

1. Hit jam shots directly at your opponent's body.
2. A jam shot is hit with the same stroke as a pass shot, except that it is hit hard in order to force a reaction shot.
3. Use this technique as a surprise, a change of pace, or to "handcuff" a quick opponent.

Jam shot

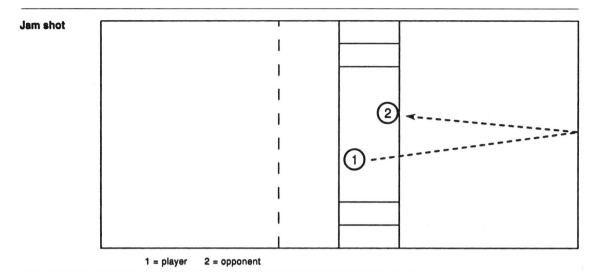

1 = player   2 = opponent

Use of the Jam Shot

When to use the jam shot:

1. As a change of pace—a surprise tactic meant to keep your opponent out of rhythm.

2. When playing a tall player. It will take him or her longer to tuck in those long limbs in order to block a jam shot.

3. When playing a quick-footed player. Hitting a ball right at the body counteracts his or her strong point—running.

Summary

1. Offensive shots mean playing to win, while defensive shots mean playing to not lose.

2. The basic offensive shots are:
   - Kill shot—A shot hit very low on the front wall
   - Pinch shot—A kill shot that hits the front and side walls near their juncture
   - Pass shot—A shot that passes an opponent and ends up in the back court

3. Kill shots and pass shots move opponents from side to side.

4. Pinch shots move opponents up; ceiling balls move them back.

5. Contact height for the kill shot is mid-calf; for a pass shot it is mid-thigh.

6. Shot selection should depend on each player's scoring zone (a spot from where a player can be consistently successful with a shot).

7. Shot selection depends on the positions of the ball and the opponent.

8. Advanced players often use the lower-percentage overhead shots as an offensive weapon.

9. The jam shot is hit hard, directly at an opponent.

8 *Backwall Play*

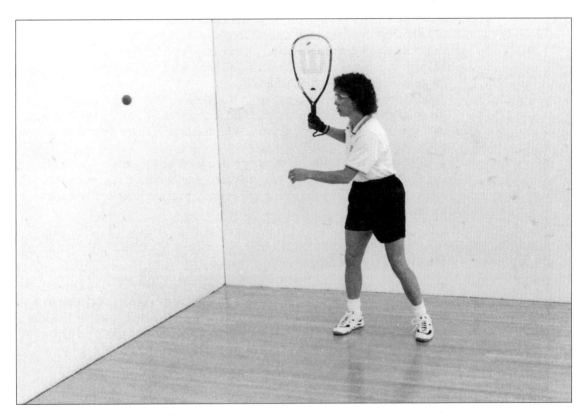

Outline

The *back wall* plays such a dominant role in racquetball that it can make or break a player's game. Close to half of the shots played in a match hit the back wall, so it is a very important aspect of becoming a competitive racquetball player.

The back wall of a racquetball court is the main feature that makes the game unique. Because of the back wall, players have to learn to deal with a ball that is traveling away from them. In most racquet sports (tennis, badminton, etc.), the ball moves only toward players, however, the backwall type of ball movement is foreign to most sports, and creates the most difficulties for beginning and intermediate players. Once one is familiar with it, however, playing balls that rebound from the back wall is a frequently used skill, especially at the beginning and intermediate levels.

Such shots should be the easiest to play because the forward movement of the ball provides much of its momentum and power. The back wall then stops the flight of the ball, slows it down a little, and sends it back toward its ultimate destination—the front wall.

As soon as a player learns the proper footwork and techniques to judge where the ball will eventually drop, the fear or intimidation caused by the back wall will disappear, and he or she will actually begin to look for that back wall set up.

Backwall Technique

In learning the *techniques* for the backwall game, it is important to remember to be patient and not rush the shot. Wait for the ball to get to a position in front of your body and drop into the desired contact zone. Actually, the ball should pass the body twice—once on its way to the back wall and again on its way to the front wall before the shot is attempted.

Footwork

The correct *footwork* for the backwall shot is the step-together-step shuffle. Begin by standing at the back wall, facing the side wall. Take a sideway step toward the front wall with your lead foot, then bring your back foot up, close to your front foot (the *step-together*). After bringing the rear foot forward, your weight should now be planted on it, in anticipation of taking the diagonal stride with your front foot into the ball (the last part of the step-together-step), just as in the forehand and backhand strokes.

Often the step-together-step motion will have to be repeated, as the ball may rebound farther forward, depending on how hard it has been hit.

One backwall skill that must be learned by all players is the ability to glide smoothly all the way to the front wall. Avoid crossing your feet (a common error in backwall play), which can cause tangled feet and an embarrassing fall, or shots taken with the weight on the wrong foot. Practice the step-together-step motion until it results in a smooth glide. Regardless of the number of times this motion is repeated, it should always end with a diagonal step into the ball.

Backwall play
Contact points for ball: (A) with opponent's racquet, (B) with front wall, (C) with floor, (D) passes player first time, (E) contacts back wall (F) passes player second time

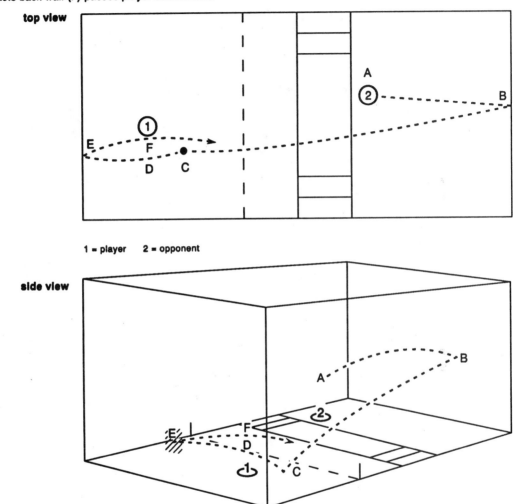

top view

1 = player   2 = opponent

side view

The last step is the same as in the backhand and forehand strokes. Plant the back foot, step diagonally with the front foot, wait for the ball to pass your body, then hit the ball. In backwall play, it's step-together, plant the back foot, and make the final step into the ball.

The Stroke

The *stroke* used when playing a ball that rebounds from the back wall is the same as the forehand and backhand strokes, discussed in Chapters 3 and 4.

Backwall play (forehand)

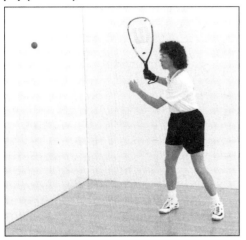

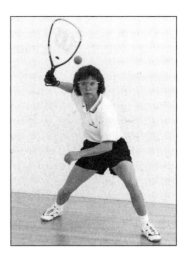

a. Ball bounces from wall, player prepares to swing   b. Backswing

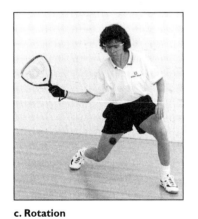

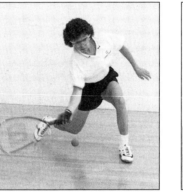

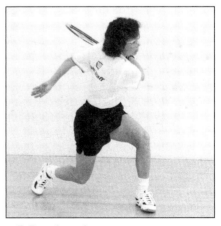

c. Rotation   d. Step forward and swing   e. Contact

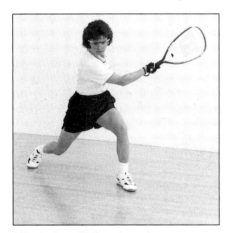

f. Beginning of follow-through   g. Follow-through

Backwall play (backhand)

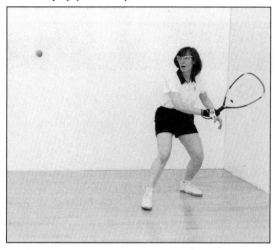

a. Ball heads to back wall

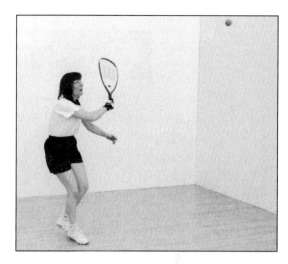

b. Passes player once and hits back wall

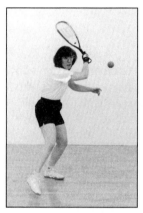

c. Player begins to swing as ball begins to come back

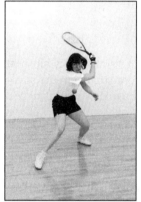

d. Player steps forward

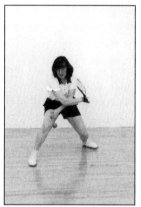

e. Lowers racquet head

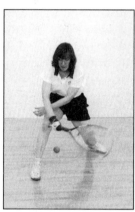

f. Rotates

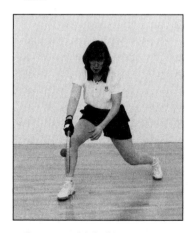

g. Contacts with ball

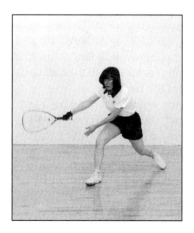

h. Begins follow-through

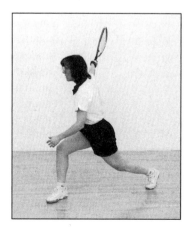

i. Finishes follow-through

Checklist for Backwall Technique

1. Face the side wall.
2. Have your racquet in the backswing position.
3. Use the step-together-step shuffle to move up to a position slightly behind the ball.
4. Do not cross your feet.
5. Wait until the ball passes your body on its way to the front wall before beginning the stroke.
6. Allow the ball to drop to the desired contact point below your knee before hitting it.
7. When the ball is near your front foot, stride diagonally into the ball and begin a full swing with your arm extended, following through completely.

The Key

The *key* to hitting solid and consistent backwall shots is to be patient and allow the ball to pass your body before you begin the stroke. This provides you with a position behind the shot and enables you to take a forward step into the ball.

This is crucial to successful backwall play. Allow the ball to pass your body first before making contact with the ball on its way to the front wall, so that you are behind the shot.

Distance-Judging Techniques

Judging how far the ball will rebound after making contact with the back wall can be learned only through on-the-court experience.

One technique to speed up this learning process is to use the step-together-step method to get to an area halfway between the anticipated landing spot and the back wall. This will allow the ball to pass your body on its way to the front wall and permit you to take a full stride into it. Beginners usually take a position near the point where the ball lands, causing them to hit the ball behind the midpoint of the body.

One common error is planting both feet and waiting for the ball. Once both feet are planted, the ball is in control instead of the player. If an error has been made in judging the spot where the ball will land, or if it takes an odd bounce, the player may find it very difficult to make an adjustment. Step-together-step puts the shooter in control of the ball, not the ball in control of the shot.

Moving back and then forward with the path of the ball allows for a margin of error in judgment of where the ball will land. If you make such an error, you can make adjustments in your direction as long as your feet are moving. It is better to go too deep in the court than not deep enough, because it is easier and quicker to move forward than backward. Also, not going far enough back

Checklist for Distance-Judging Techniques

1. Position yourself halfway between the spot where the ball will land and the back wall.
2. Stay far enough behind the ball so you can stride into it after it passes your body.
3. If a ball is hit high and slow, take a position as near the back wall as possible.
4. If a ball is hit low and hard, take a position near the service zone.
5. Stay behind the ball—it is easier to move forward than backward.
6. Use the step-together-step shuffle; avoid planting your feet.

will probably mean that the ball will have to be played near your rear foot instead of your front foot.

The exception to going to the back of the court would be when the ball is hit very hard and rebounds to a position in front of your body, or if the ball makes contact with the back wall on the fly. In these cases, remain in center court, wait for the ball to pass, and use proper footwork and the correct stroke.

The speed and the height at which the ball is traveling will give a clue as to how far the ball will rebound. A ball hit slowly and high on the front wall will not rebound very far from the back wall. In this case, the best position will be as near to the back wall as possible, permitting forward movement with the ball. If a ball is hit with power and at a low to medium height, it will rebound farther from the back wall, requiring you to be positioned farther from the back wall.

There is no substitute for experience. Practice and experiment in order to learn how to judge backwall shots. Mastering these skills can eliminate the fear of backwall play and elicit eager anticipation of a backwall set up.

Summary

1. Backwall play makes racquetball unique among racquet sports.
2. A large percentage of balls rebound from the back wall.
3. Beginners often have trouble judging how far the ball will rebound and lack confidence in their ability to do well in backwall play.
4. Learning the step-together-step shuffle can help a player develop confidence in backwall skills.
5. It is important to take a position behind the landing point of the ball, in order to be able to stride into the ball.
6. Common errors include planting the feet, crossing the feet, hitting the ball near the rear foot, not getting deep enough, and making rebound-judgment errors.
7. The speed and height of the shot determine how far the ball will rebound from the back wall.

9 *The Service Game*

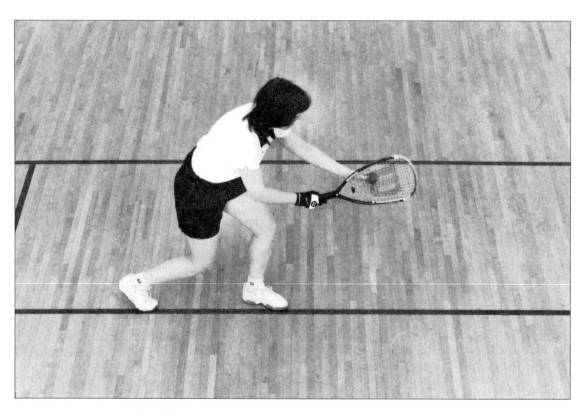

Outline

Once the basic strokes and strategies are mastered, the *service* becomes the most important part of racquetball. It is the only time a player can stand in a specific, chosen spot on the court, place the ball in a selected position, and know where the opponent is located. Also, the server is the only player who can score on a rally. It is important to take advantage of this unique situation and develop a strong service game, so you can use this major weapon in a positive manner.

While a wide variety of serves may exist, there are three basic serves that are necessary to a good service game. These basic serves are: the drive serve, the "Z" serve, and the lob serve. You can change height, speed, and angle of contact of these serves to provide yourself with an almost unlimited selection.

The Drive Serve

The *drive serve* is a low, hard serve. The goal of a drive serve is to have the ball bounce twice before reaching the back wall. It should be directed toward one of the rear corners, restricting an opponent to a weak return. Since the server can utilize the entire service zone, the best position in which to begin is with the back foot on the short line (the back line of the service zone). This allows the server to stride forward and use the entire service zone to utilize the full force of the body. The server may stand on this line, but not cross over into the rear court area.

Since the serve is made with a forehand motion, the server will use the same stride, swing, and follow-through explained in Chapter 3. Make certain that the ball is dropped far enough forward and out to the side to allow you to make a full swing. Step forward with authority, point your forward foot toward a front corner of the court, and strike the ball with maximum power on its downward flight. Be certain to bend at the knees instead of the waist, and keep both eyes on the ball while executing a smooth forehand stroke. The contact point should be low enough to make the ball rebound from the front wall and strike the floor just past the short service line as it heads for a rear corner. If

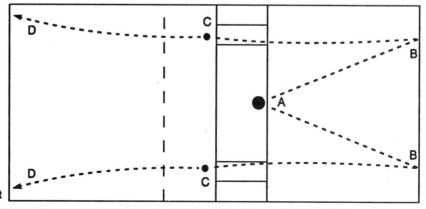

Drive Serve (2 shots)

Contact points for ball:
(A) with racquet
(B) with front wall
(C) with floor
(D) deep into back court

Checklist for the Drive Serve

1. Stand deep in the service zone, with your knees slightly bent.
2. Drop the ball far ahead and out to the side.
3. Take a full stride into the ball.
4. Keep your head down and your eyes focused on the ball.
5. Wait for the ball to drop into the contact zone.
6. Hit the ball hard with a full forehand stroke and complete the follow through.
7. Hit the ball hard and low enough to make it land just past the short service line.
8. With a proper serve, the ball will bounce twice before it hits the rear corner.

the serve is executed properly, the ball will bounce again before striking the back wall, making it difficult, if not impossible, for an opponent to return.

The "Z" Serve

The "Z" serve may be used from either the left or right side of the service zone. The ball is hit toward the opposite front corner, hitting the front wall then the side wall. This causes the ball to travel toward the opposite rear corner (see diagram below). A well-executed "Z" serve will cross the service zone and bounce in the rear court before making contact with the side wall at a point near the back wall. The ball will then travel parallel to the back wall. (Note that the ball should not hit the back wall.)

"Z" serve

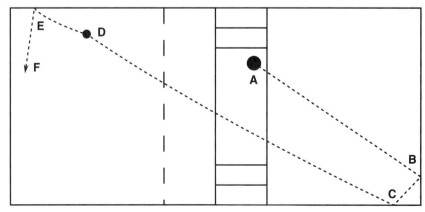

Contact points for ball:
(A) with racquet
(B) with front wall
(C) with side wall
(D) with floor
(E) with second side wall
(F) continues into
    back court

Checklist for the "Z" Serve

1. To make a "Z" serve, stand on one side of the service zone.
2. The "Z" serve hits the front wall first, then the side wall.
3. After bouncing, the ball should hit the second side wall before making contact with the back wall.
4. The ball should "jump" from the side wall, parallel to the back wall.
5. Avoid letting the ball hit the back wall.
6. Hitting the front wall close to the side wall provides more rotation, resulting in the ball traveling parallel to the back wall.
7. Hitting the front wall farther from the side wall gives the ball a wider "Z" path, causing it to strike the back wall.
8. Change speeds to add variety.

The closer the ball is hit to the front corner, the more rotation it will pick up, making it bounce or "jump" farther off the side wall, deep in the back court. The farther the ball hits from the front corner, the more it will travel in a wide "Z" pattern, resulting in the ball rolling off the side wall and making contact with the back wall, instead of jumping off the side wall parallel to the back wall.

By varying velocity from hard drive to soft lob, you can give the "Z" serve a variety of looks, thus preventing the opponent from cheating to one side or the other to cut off your serve before it hits the side wall.

The Lob Serve

The *lob serve* is rapidly becoming the most popular serve in racquetball. Once used only as a second serve, the lob is now often used as a first serve. With the advent of faster balls and oversized, graphite racquets, players find it difficult to keep drive and "Z" serves from rebounding off the back wall, which provides opponents with easy set ups. The lob serve is a good solution to this situation.

The lob serve does three things for the service game. First, it allows the server to get into the rally without giving the receiver an opportunity to make an offensive shot. Second, it sometimes tempts opponents into attempting a low-percentage offensive shot, which then gives the server a set up for an immediate winning point. Third, the serve attacks a very weak area of the receiver's stroke—the chest area or above.

In hitting the lob serve, the goal is to get the ball to bounce high into either rear corner of the court. This serve is an exception to most racquetball shots, in that the wrist is not used; the lob is a slow, deliberate stroke. The ball should

**Three lob serves
(top view)**

a. Basic lob serve

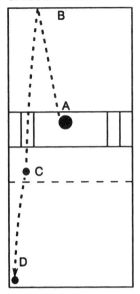

Contact points for ball:
(A) with racquet
(B) with front wall
(C) with floor
(D) with floor deep in
     back court

b. Angle lob serve

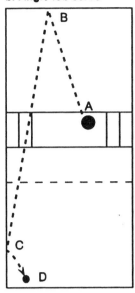

Contact points for ball:
(A) with racquet
(B) with front wall
(C) with side wall
(D) with floor

c. Z-lob serve

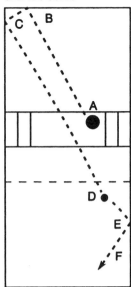

Contact points for ball:
(A) with racquet
(B) with front wall
(C) with side wall
(D) with floor
(E) with second side wall
(F) continues toward
     back wall

**Three lob serves
(angled view)**

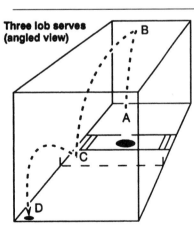

a. Basic lob serve
Contact points for ball:
(A) with racquet
(B) with front wall
(C) with floor in center court
(D) with floor in deep court

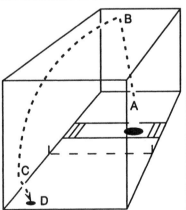

b. Angle lob serve
Contact points for ball:
(A) with racquet
(B) with front wall
(C) with side wall
(D) with floor

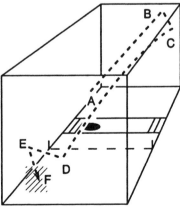

c. Z-lob serve
Contact points for ball:
(A) with racquet
(B) with front wall
(C) with side wall
(D) with floor
(E) with second side wall
(F) continues toward back wall

Checklist for the Lob Serve

1. Hit the lob serve with a stiff wrist and a slow, soft, deliberate stroke.
2. The ball should make contact with the front wall as high as possible.
3. The ball should land in the five-foot safety zone.
4. The ball should bounce in a high arc.
5. The ball should bounce high in a rear corner.
6. The lob serve should force your opponent into an above-the-shoulder return.

be hit with a sidearm, scooping motion and should contact on the front wall as high as possible without hitting the ceiling. The ensuing bounce will be high enough to force an opponent to return the serve above waist level.

By changing the front wall contact point, you can create a variety of lob serves. The first type of lob is the bread and butter, or basic, lob serve. You can hit this lob to either side of the court from anywhere in the service zone. The ball should travel in a high arc and land in the first five feet behind the rear line of the service zone. This area is the safety zone, which your opponent may not enter to cut off a serve. After this first bounce, the ball will make another high arc in the corner of the court, forcing your opponent to hit the ball above shoulder level.

Another type of lob serve is similar to the basic lob except that the ball hits the front wall at an angle, causing it to make contact high on the side wall, close to the back wall. This serve creates an angle that jams the opponent, making it difficult for him or her to get arm extension.

Still another variety of the lob serve, the "Z" lob, is hit very high into either corner of the front wall. It follows the same path as a "Z" serve, leaving your opponent with a difficult return because the ball bounces high and toward the side wall.

The Jam Serve

The *jam serve* is a secondary serve, to be used after establishing the drive serve as a potent weapon. Hit with the same motion as a drive serve, it can keep your opponent off balance. Instead of aiming the ball directly at a rear corner, when attempting the jam serve you should try to make the ball hit a side wall and then rebound toward the feet of the receiver.

The jam serve hits the front wall slightly higher than the drive serve, makes contact with the side wall even with the server's body, and lands near the receiver's feet, which results in a jamming effect.

This serve is effective if the receiver is anticipating a drive serve and is moving to a corner, and is even more effective when used to jam the opponent on the backhand side. It may be served from anywhere in the service zone.

Jam serve

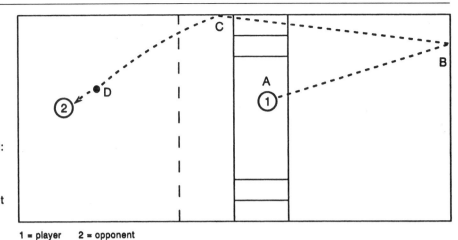

Contact points for ball:
(A) with racquet
(B) with front wall
(C) with side wall
(D) with floor near feet
of opponent

1 = player   2 = opponent

✓ *Checklist for the Jam Serve*

1. The service motion should resemble that used in the drive serve.
2. The ball should make contact with the side wall and rebound at the receiver's feet.
3. Use this serve when the receiver is anticipating a drive serve.
4. Develop a strong drive serve before attempting the jam serve.

The Theory of Deceptive Serving

Variety is the key to successful serving in racquetball. Most players begin while standing in the middle of the service zone, opening with a drive serve to the opponent's backhand. If that misses, they then hit a lob serve to the backhand as their second serve. This sets up a predictable pattern, giving receivers the chance to know what serve to expect and plan how to return it.

Avoid being predictable in your serving pattern. Variety permits the server to score points even when hitting a poor serve, because the receiver doesn't know what serve to expect. This gives the server a great psychological advantage. One way to accomplish this is by what is called *deceptive serving,* a means to keep the receiver off balance and guessing.

Deceptive serving depends on the server's ability to deliver a variety of serves from at least four areas of the service zone; that is, being able to execute at least four serves from four different spots.

From the left side of the service zone, a server can hit a drive serve to the backhand and forehand, a "Z" serve to the backhand, and jam and lob serves to both sides.

Four positions for deceptive serving with four service paths for each position

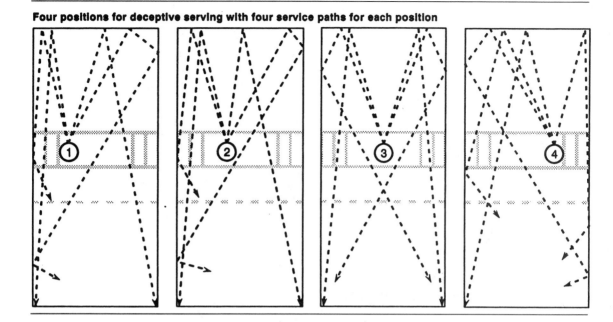

✓	*Checklist for the Deceptive Serving*

1. Variety is the key.
2. Be unpredictable.
3. Learn to serve from four areas in the service zone.
4. Master at least four serves from each area.

The same options are available from the area between the left position and the center of the service zone, but the angle and presentation are different, which forces the receiver to make adjustments to the return.

One should also be able to take some of the velocity off of a drive serve or "Z" serve and make it slower. (This is just like a baseball pitcher throwing a changeup.) This maneuver can create a whole new set of problems for the opponent, by upsetting his or her timing, footwork, and stroke.

The options from the center of the court are limited only by the skill of the server. Players at all skill levels should be able to hit drive serves and lob serves to both the forehand and backhand, and as skill levels progress, "Z" serves to the forehand and backhand can be added.

From the right side of the court, drives and lobs to both sides and a "Z" serve to the forehand side are at the server's disposal.

With a deceptive serving strategy, there can be as many as twenty different serves with which to baffle a confused receiver. If the server is constantly changing serving position and types of serves, the receiver cannot anticipate what serve to expect. This freezes the opponent in the ready position and inter-feres with any movement or "cheating" before the ball is seen in flight. Deceptive serving offers a much better attack than the traditional drive serve–lob serve strategy.

Remember: While serving, the server is in total control, the only player to know what kind of serve will be next and to where the ball will be aimed. The rules allow the server ten seconds in which to serve the ball. There is no need to hurry or rush. Take as much time as you need to concentrate on and visual-ize your chosen serve before actually beginning it. Deceptive serving can help the server control the match and score the points needed to win.

Summary

1. Other than mastering the basic strokes, the service game is the most important part of racquetball.
2. It is important to master the basic serves from various areas of the service zone and with different speeds.
3. Serves fall into three main categories:
   - Drive serves
   - "Z" serves
   - Lob serves
4. The drive serve is the basic serve. An opponent's anticipation of it makes the other serves effective.
5. The drive serve is hit low and hard into one of the rear corners.
6. The "Z" serve uses all of the walls and can be confusing to an opponent.
7. The lob serve is hit softly and high on the front wall in order to make it bounce high enough to force a shoulder-high return.
8. The jam serve is effective because it mimics a drive serve and rebounds suddenly, directly at the receiver's feet.

10 *Service Returns*

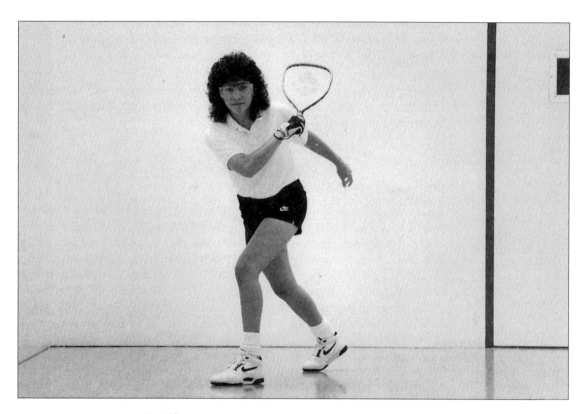

Outline

A breakdown of the important points of the service return process includes shot selection and the strategy behind it, correct footwork, and the mental aspect of service returns.

The receiver of a serve is in a position to either lose a point or to gain control of center court. Thus the two aims of a receiver are to keep the ball in play and regain center court position.

Remember the two basic rules of receiving:

1. Do not skip the ball; make your opponent earn the point in a rally.

2. Get the server out of center court and take control of that position.

This does not mean that the receiver should never attempt a kill shot, but doing so should be of lower priority, due to the risk of giving the server an easy, uncontested point. Only attempt a kill shot on a service return if the serve is a perfect set up, or if the server leaves an average set up but backs too far out of the service zone after serving the ball.

The Ceiling Ball Return

Most successful players prefer to get into a rally with good center court position. Two ways to accomplish this are to return with a ceiling ball or a pass shot. The *ceiling ball return* is a high-percentage shot that forces the server into deep court, leaving the center area so it can be taken over by the receiver. The ball should be directed into one of the rear corners, forcing an opponent hitting a return to battle the angle formed by the corner of the walls.

It is important to keep the ceiling ball from hitting the side wall, coming up short, or rebounding from the back wall. Ideally, the ceiling return will make your opponent play the shot with a return from above the waist. (It is difficult to hit a good offensive shot from this position.)

The goal of the ceiling return is to create a situation that forces the server to hit an above-the-waist return from deep in the court, thus allowing the receiver to take control of center court position.

The Pass Shot Return

When hit properly, the *pass shot return* should force a side out or a weak return. As with the ceiling return, try to direct pass shots toward one of the rear corners. The pass shot return will also move the server out of center court. The receiver's margin of error with this shot is smaller than with the ceiling ball return.

When hitting a pass shot, be sure your point of contact is at hip level or below. This should keep the ball from bouncing off the back wall and creating an easy set up for your opponent.

Immediately after hitting the pass shot, quickly run to center court and take a position to prepare for the next shot.

Ceiling ball return (2 shots)

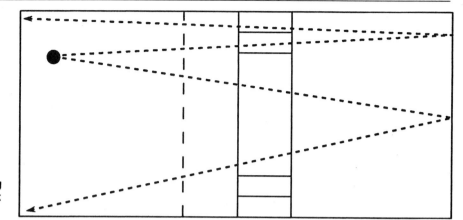

a. Top view showing target zones in back court

b. Side view showing path of each ball
Contact points for ball:
(A) with racquet
(B) with ceiling
(C) with front wall
(D) with floor
(E) with floor in deep court

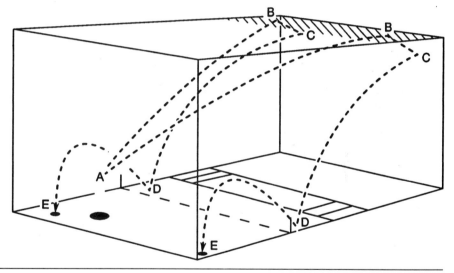

Return Selection

The main criteria in determining which return to select—ceiling, pass, or kill—are the type, direction, and velocity of the serve. As a general rule of thumb, remember these three points:

1. When the serve is not an easy set up, hit a ceiling ball return. If the serve does not set you up, it may mean fighting a tough, corner serve, one hit close into the body, or one that somehow surprises you. If you are unsure as to what kind of return to use (even if you are set up), *go to the ceiling,* move into center court, and position yourself to attack at the next opportunity.

2. If the serve is a "semi-set up," the options are a pass shot, ceiling ball, or possibly a kill shot—depending on your capabilities. If the ball is set up and you are in position to take a full swing and control the shot, go for the pass

**Pass shot return
(2 shots)**

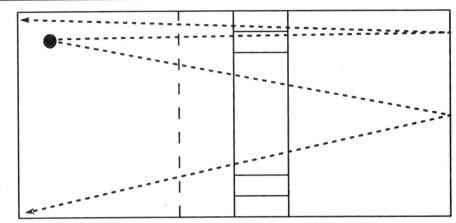

**a. Top view showing
target zones in back
court**

**b. Side view showing
path of each ball**
Contact points for ball:
(A) with racquet
(B) with front wall
(C) with floor
(D) with floor in
    deep court

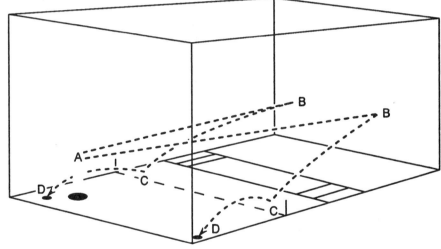

shot or kill shot. They force a quicker reaction from the opponent and often lead to a side out or weak return. As soon as you hit the shot move quickly to the center court position, because the return of your pass shot will arrive much sooner than a return from a ceiling ball.

3. If the serve is an ultimate set up, the choices are between a pass shot and a kill shot. The pass shot is the safer of the two, but the kill shot is a potential rally ender. Be warned, though, that even if the kill shot could be a rally ender, it may end the rally by giving a point to the server. When your opponent is serving, any ball you skip results in an immediate lost point, which is quite different than the side out that results when the server makes an error. Whenever you choose a kill shot as a service return, be certain to be set up mentally as well as physically. Also, be certain that you are able to execute a full swing.

Receiving Position

After discussing the types of returns, it is important to concentrate on the *positioning* and *footwork* needed for a receiver to be ready to return low, hard serves from tough opponents.

Although all service returns are important, the focus of this section will be on returning hard serves that require quick reaction: the drive, "Z," and jam serves.

When preparing to receive a serve, take a position in the middle of the court, four or five feet from the back wall. Starting too far forward leaves you vulnerable to deep drive serves into the corners, while positioning yourself too deep makes you vulnerable to hard, low, drive serves that land just past the service line. Hence, you should stand in the middle of the court. "Cheating" one way or the other leaves you open for serves to the far side. For example, a player who compensates by standing too close to the backhand side of a wall gives an alert opponent the opportunity to take advantage of the open space on the forehand side of the court.

Ready Position

The *ready position* for receiving serves is with feet spread apart a little wider than the shoulders, knees slightly bent, and weight on the balls of the feet. Avoid standing flat-footed, because it will make you need to take an extra step to get your weight onto your toes. Keep your eyes on the ball instead of the server, and be mentally ready to move quickly in any direction.

The racquet should be held loosely at the center of your body with the backhand grip, since a majority of serves will be directed toward your backhand. The top of the racquet should be pointing at the front wall, so that the strings are facing the side walls. This will make it easier to get the racquet into the backswing position (forehand or backhand). Keeping the racquet in this centered position requires only a slight lift of your shoulder to place your arm and the racquet in the forehand or backhand position.

Footwork

Footwork for returning serves is very simple, but a great number of players execute it incorrectly.

The first step is the one that many players get wrong. It should be a crossover step toward the direction of the ball. If the serve is to the left, step with the right foot first, crossing over the left foot; if the ball is hit to the right, step with the left foot crossing over the right. The error made by many players is to first step with the foot closest to the ball and then cross over. This extra step does not add power or improve balance and slows the time it takes to get into the backswing position and to the ball. Learning to eliminate this extra step will enable you to get to the ball quicker and in a position ready to hit the ball.

Ready position for service return

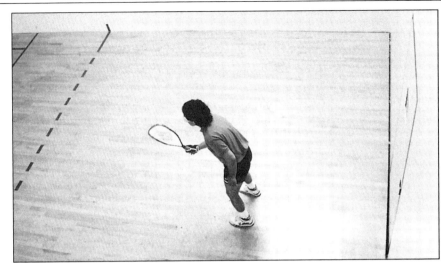

a. Correct

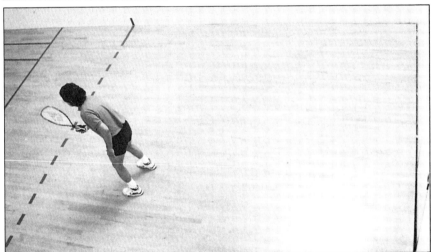

b. Incorrect:
   too far forward

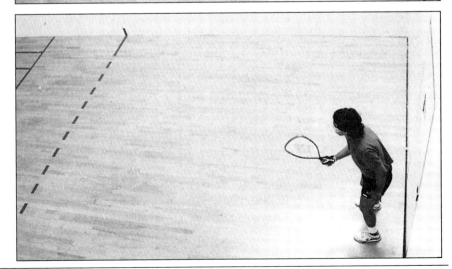

c. Incorrect:
   too far back

Service return footwork (backhand)

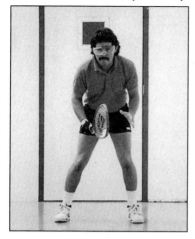

a. Ready

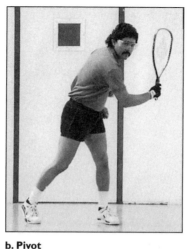

b. Pivot

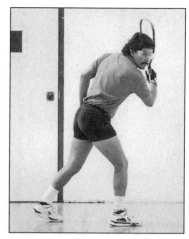

c. Cross-over step

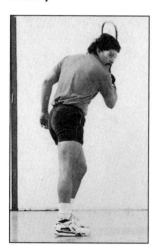

d. Plant back foot

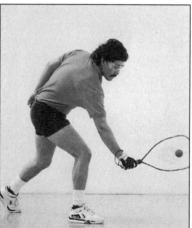

e. Contact

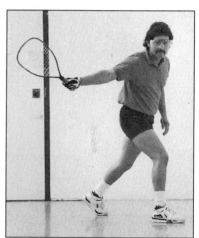

f. Follow-through

After this crossover step, the trailing foot replants, followed by a step into the ball. Once the crossover step is accomplished, one can shuffle to the point of impact, if necessary. The planted back foot allows adjustments to be made to aid balance and generate more power and thrust while stepping into the shot. At this point the racquet should be approaching the backswing position.

The Mental Aspect of Service Return

The physical aspect of service return is very important, but there *is* another side—the mental. Among things to be considered are the score, how well you

Service return footwork (forehand)

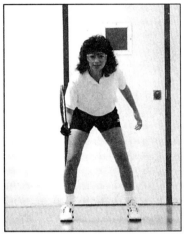

a. Ready

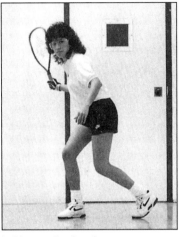

b. Pivot to forehand

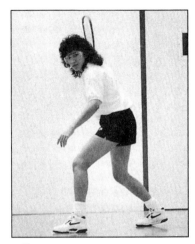

c. Cross-over step

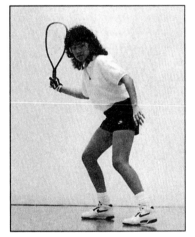

d. Plant back foot

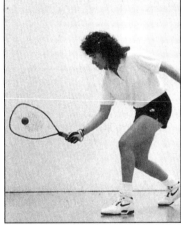

e. Contact

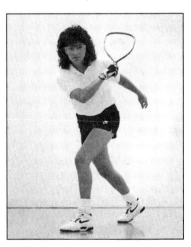

f. Follow-through

are playing, the momentum of the game, the skills of the server, and physical condition of both players.

One question is when to go for that 40-foot kill shot. (Probably not at match point or 10–10 in a tie-breaker.) Remember: the attempted rally-ending kill shot can also end the game in the opponent's favor. It's like hitting a three-run home run in the bottom of the ninth—it can happen, but not very often.

A better time to try a lower-percentage shot is when the score is in your favor, or if it is still early in the match. As the match continues and the score remains close, choose higher-percentage shots, giving the opponent an opportunity to make some errors.

Checklist for Service Returns

1. Take the ready position in the midline of the court, about three-quarters of the way from the short line or four or five feet from the back wall.
2. Keep your eyes on the ball instead of the server.
3. Ceiling balls and pass shots are the most common types of returns.
4. The first step to either side should be a crossover step.
5. The goal of the return is to force the server out of the center court area and take that position for yourself.
6. Keep ceiling shots from hitting the back wall, forcing the server to play them from above the waist.
7. Hit pass shots and ceiling shots into one of the rear corners.
8. Move to center court position immediately after hitting a ceiling or pass return.
9. Be aware of the game situation when determining shot selection.
10. Analyze your opponent's style, looking for changes.

Continue to evaluate yourself and your opponent during the match. Changes will usually occur. Quick players may not always be quick and defensive players don't always play consistent defense.

When a quick opponent is tired, be more aggressive on service returns. Drive the ball to force a quick reaction, which will be difficult for a tired player. If your opponent recovers and begins reaching aggressive returns, revert to a patient style of return.

Sometimes a defensive player will have a hot streak and shoot everything for winners, scoring point after point. In such a situation, your defensive-minded opponent has become an aggressive player; this may be the time to become a defensive player yourself and hit defensive shots to the normally defensive player.

By constantly analyzing and evaluating the current situation, learn to make whatever adjustments in your service returns that are necessary to win the match. Continue analyzing your opponent, but realize that what you are evaluating can change. Make adjustments, and do whatever you think will help you to maintain control and keep your opponent off balance.

When playing well, an opponent will probably want to serve immediately after each rally to maintain his or her rhythm and momentum. You can slow the game down by using the full time allowed to receive the serve (10 seconds), or by returning serves with ceiling balls, forcing the server to play defensively or to attempt low-percentage offensive shots. Conversely, if an opponent is playing poorly and missing shots, you should utilize serves that will encourage weak shots by your opponent, giving you set ups.

The service return is the first opportunity for the receiver to take control of the rally. Use good judgment and good footwork and always be aware of the game situation. This will get you into the serving box more often and force your opponent to be the one to play service returns.

Summary

1. Service returns are an important part of racquetball because the receiver of a serve is in an immediate position to lose a point, while the server can only lose service.
2. The receiver should be sure that the ball hits the front wall, so the server will have to win a rally for a point instead of scoring an ace.
3. The receiver should try to get the server out of center court and take control of that position.
4. Ceiling and passing returns are designed to move the server into deep court and allow the receiver to take control of center position.
5. Type, direction, and velocity of serves determine which return is best to use.
6. A crossover on the first step in either direction will help the receiver get into position to return the serve more quickly.
7. The mental aspect of the service game includes analyzing the score, the game's momentum, and both players' skills and physical condition.
8. The way the game is played may change as the factors cited in number 7 change during the game. The smart player learns to take advantage of changing game situations.

11   *Developing a Winning Strategy*

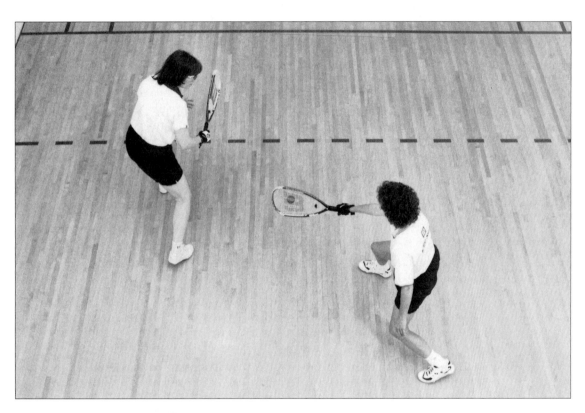

Outline

As one becomes more adept at the skills of racquetball, it is important to play increasingly difficult opponents. This competition may be found in a class, a recreational game, or an organized or sanctioned tournament. Developing an effective game strategy is important in each game of racquetball. The mind must know what it is trying to accomplish so that the body can perform effectively.

Analyzing an Opponent

While warming up, analyze the strengths and weaknesses of your opponent. Which tendencies can you defeat? Which areas and shots should be avoided in your game plan? Here are a couple of examples of opponent analysis:

- *Watching your opponent's stroke during the warm up*—Watch the drop and hit stroke. Is it hit hard? Does it seem erratic? Is the ball contacted too close to the body? Is your opponent's weight on the back foot when hitting?

- *When rallying*—Are the opponent's shots consistent or are they hit sometimes early, sometimes late, sometimes too close or too far from the body?

A smart player will look for keys to a prospective opponent's style of play. When preparing to play an opponent, look to see if the player:

- Hits the ball when it is behind him or her. (Such players tend to hit pinch shots rather than straight kills.)

- Lets the ball get too close to the body. (Such players do more pushing and generally more pinching than stroking.)

- Hits the ball in front of the body. (Such players usually hit cross-court effectively.)

- Shows no rhythm or method to his or her stroke patterns. (Such players must continue to be watched if you are to find keys to their game.)

- Shows a preference for one side of the body. (If a player hits fewer backhands during the warm up, challenge his or her backhand early in the match.)

Another key is how the player warms up. The sluggish player will tend to stay with the drop and hit shots, while the aggressive player will move a great deal in order to warm up the legs as well as the arms and shoulders.

Also look for glaring weaknesses:

- Hitting ceiling balls. (Serve more lob serves and hit ceiling balls during rallies, to force ceiling returns.)

- Limited variety of serves or a definite pattern. (This allows you to anticipate.)

- Ability to move to one side of the court better than to the other side.

- Handles back wall or side wall shots poorly.

Look for other keys by noting physical characteristics: quick hands; fast or slow; on the toes or flat-footed; or inconsistent strokes.

In each game, develop a strategy that will take away an opponent's strengths and take advantage of his or her weaknesses. Slow the pace with ceiling balls for an aggressive player and speed up the attacking part of your

Checklist for Analyzing an Opponent

1. Look for strengths and weaknesses.
2. Look for errors in footwork, stride, stroke, contact point, and follow-through.
3. Look for tendencies to emphasize certain strokes or aspects of the game.
4. Look for tendencies in service patterns.
5. Take note of physical traits and style of play.
6. Plan to take away opportunities for your opponent to employ strengths, and take advantage of weaknesses.

game against a defensive player. Make a slow player move and hit directly at a mobile player. It is important to know your opponent's favorite shot. This is the shot to take away and to be ready to handle.

Strategy Against Different Types of Players

As your court time increases, you will notice how most players tend to fit into specific categories; the sprinter, or hustler, who seems to get to every shot; the tall, lanky player, who can almost touch both side walls without moving; the stationary player, who controls center court; the power hitter; and the patient player, who frustrates opponents. Following are analyses of these categories.

The Rabbit

The *rabbit* is the quick player who gets to every shot. This type of player likes to run. Because this player's strength is speed, turn this speed into defeat by hitting shots directly at the rabbit's position after the last return, or by slowing the pace of the game with lob shots or ceiling balls.

For example, assume that both players are on the left side of the court. The rabbit will usually run to the right side. Hit the ball to where the rabbit was standing. Having to stand and wait for the shot can drive the rabbit crazy. Usually this player hits very well on the run but not too well when he or she is standing still. So when playing the rabbit, hit slow, seemingly plum set ups. This can destroy his or her timing.

Checklist for the Rabbit

1. Hit balls directly at the speedy player (the rabbit).
2. Emphasize lobs and ceiling balls.
3. Try to slow the pace.
4. Try to keep the rabbit in one spot.

Checklist for the Giraffe

1. Hit jamming shots at the tall, lanky player (the giraffe).
2. Hit pinch shots.
3. Avoid passing shots.
4. Try to force the giraffe to move forward and then back.

The Giraffe

The *giraffe* is the tall player with long arms. This type of player prefers to stay in the center of the court and get every shot as it comes by. Passing shots are not good choices against the giraffe. Hit the ball right at the center of that lanky body in a "jamming" manner.

While he or she usually possesses a quick first step, the giraffe is usually not quick enough to move forward and backward effectively. Hit pinch shots that force such a player to move forward to the front of the court, immediately followed by shots to force movement back, deep in the court.

The Slug

The *slug* is rather slow but, when allowed to set up, can hit good strokes and put the ball wherever he or she desires.

Although slow, the slug usually anticipates well. Get him or her moving. Pinch shots are an important tool against this type of player. It is essential to make the slug move forward and back. A pinch shot, even if it is a little high, will force the slug to run.

Another good choice is a "V" pass. When the slug is in center court, the "V" pass will hit the front wall, the side wall, then cut in behind the opponent. It makes the slug spin, turn, and run.

The Peacock or Poser

The *peacock* or *poser* is another common type. The peacock always wants to look good and in control. Such a player displays smooth strokes and usually will hold the follow-through position after the shot. This is why the peacock is

Checklist for the Slug

1. Hit pinch shots or "V" passes against the slow player (the slug).
2. Make the slug move forward and then backward.

Checklist for the Peacock or Poser

1. Use unorthodox shots and patterns to upset the poise and control of the poser.
2. Hit jamming shots.
3. Hit pinch shots, ceiling balls, and pass shots.
4. Try to move the peacock back into deep court.

also called a *poser*. You should try to take this facade away and make him or her look bad.

Try jamming the ball into the body. This will force a "herky-jerky" motion in order to return the ball and will take away the opportunity to make a picture-perfect stroke. Make the peacock run so there is no time for him or her to pose. Use pinch shots, ceiling balls, and pass shots to move the player back, and use unorthodox shots to create mental havoc—"Z" balls, around-the-wall balls, and other offbeat shots that can take away that feeling (and look) of control.

The Police Dog

The *police dog* is an aggressive player who likes to hit everything hard. These "runner-gunners" like to play powerful, low, fast racquetball. Lob serves, around-the-wall balls, "Z" balls, and ceiling balls can upset this game plan tremendously, so use these shots as the ultimate strategy against police dog players. These one-speed (zoom!) swingers don't like to adjust to a finesse game. Place the ball at chest height or higher to make it difficult for them to swing hard. It is a must to keep this "dog" at bay.

The Saint Bernard

Last, but not least, is the *Saint Bernard*. This type of player is just the opposite of the police dog—they want to play soft, high balls until an opponent gets fed up with the slow, finesse game. A tendency toward dump shots, slow passing

 Checklist for the Police Dog

1. Hit lob serves against the power player (the police dog).
2. Hit around-the-wall balls, "Z" balls, and ceiling balls.
3. Try to force chest-high (or higher) returns.
4. Avoid giving the police dog a chance to kill or hit hard.

Checklist for the Saint Bernard

1. Play aggressively against the finesse type of player (the Saint Bernard).
2. Emphasize hitting the ball hard.
3. Drive the ball down and hard from all positions on the court.
4. Hit low, hard serves and hard "Z" serves.

shots, and touch shots gives the Saint Bernard player an attack with all the speed of frozen maple syrup. A strategy to use against this kind of player is to be as aggressive as possible. When returning a ceiling ball, bring it down and hit it as hard as possible. Hit overhead drive shots when the ball is above your head. Drive the ball down. Keep the ball low and fast with Saint Bernard players, forcing them out of the slow, mistake-free game that is their staple. Serve low, hard drive serves and hard "Z" serves. Be aggressive and keep driving the ball.

Developing an All-Around Game

In order to be able to play against various types of players, you must develop an all-around game (the ability to hit high, slow shots and fast, low shots), but one that is uniquely your own.

Always play your style of game; don't get suckered into playing someone else's. Doing so gives your opponent the advantage, who then feels comfortable with his or her game plan. Develop your own game plan, making certain to include versatility. That way you will feel more comfortable when strategy changes occur. Find strength in the fact that you have an all-around, not a one-dimensional, game.

Summary

1. Analyze an opponent's style of play, looking for tendencies, strengths, and weaknesses.
2. Develop a game style of your own, designed to counter opponents' strong points and take advantage of their weaknesses.
3. Play different types of players. This will help you develop a versatile game, enabling you to adjust to any type of opponent strategy and counter it effectively with your own.

12   *The Three-Wall Game*

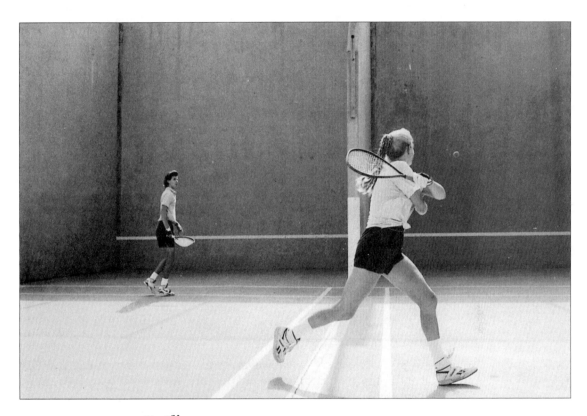

Outline

Three-wall is a popular form of racquetball that combines the challenge of a racquet sport with the advantages of playing out of doors in the sunshine and fresh air. Many three-wall facilities are found at schools and parks, especially in Western states where the winters are mild. The cost of construction and maintenance is much less than for a four-wall facility.

Many of these facilities were originally used as outdoor handball courts. The three-wall game evolved from handball, as did the indoor four-wall game.

Most of the skills are the same as in the indoor game: forehand, backhand, kill shots, pinch shots, etc. The main difference, obviously, is that there is no back wall or ceiling, eliminating the need for back wall and ceiling related shots. "Quick feet" can be a real asset in three-wall. Three-wall stresses quickness, court position, and more sidearm and overhead strokes, because once a shot passes there is no back wall or side wall to keep the ball in play. Without these walls, quick steps to reach the ball as it rebounds directly from the front wall are a necessary replacement for the court coverage of four-wall.

There are a variety of types of three-wall courts, with different side wall lengths and slants. Beginning with a minimum length of 20 feet, some side walls have a constant height of 20 feet while others taper down from the front wall to a height of 12 feet.

The court dimensions are the same as four-wall: 20 feet by 40 feet, with a 20 foot front wall. The service zone, service line, short-line, and service box are also the same.

The main difference is that there are two-inch lines that mark the limits of the three-wall playing area: side lines and a back line. The side lines are extensions of the side walls, and the rear line is 40 feet from the front wall.

Rule Differences

Three-wall is played very similarly to four-wall. All of the *rule differences* are the result of the missing surfaces or the side and rear lines.

A long serve occurs when a serve lands directly past the rear line before first touching the ground. This may be compared to a long serve that hits the back wall in four-wall—a fault serve.

An out serve unique to three-wall is one that is hit too high by the server and goes over the front wall or hits the screen that is often attached to the top of the front wall. Another out serve is one that lands wide or outside of either side line.

A rally ends when any shot that rebounds directly from a wall lands wide, outside of either side line, or behind the rear line. Scoring and general play are the same as with their indoor cousin, but the strategy and court position techniques may vary.

Court hinders may differ from court to court. Since courts are often side by side, the ball or a player from one court may wander onto a neighboring court, causing a hinder. Any time this occurs, play should immediately stop and the point should be replayed as a hinder. Loose balls and especially stray players from adjacent courts can cause a hazard to the players. A player may also call a hinder if a shot takes him or her onto a neighboring court, where the safety of another player causes his or her swing to be inhibited.

Diagram of three-wall court with measurements

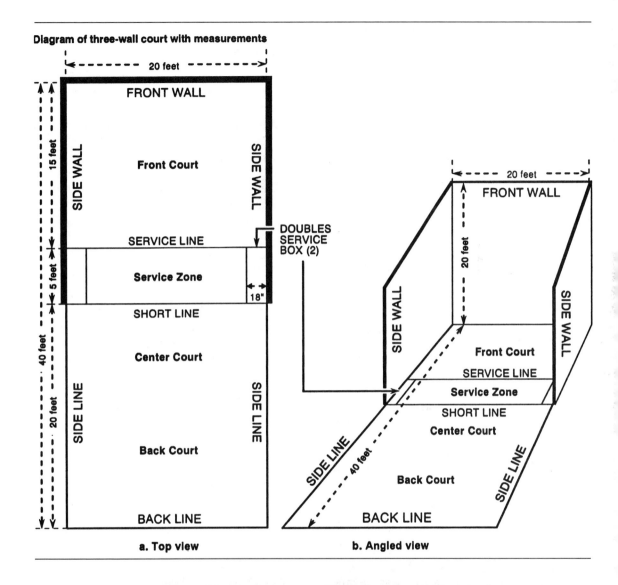

a. Top view

b. Angled view

✓ *Checklist for Rule Differences*

1. Fault serves: A long serve is when the ball first lands past the rear line.
2. Out serves: A high serve is when the ball is hit too high over the front wall surface; a wide serve occurs when the ball first lands outside of a side or rear line.
3. A rally ends if a ball lands outside of a side line before bouncing in the playing area.
4. Hinders occur whenever a player or a ball from another court enters the playing area, or when a player is forced to hold up a swing to avoid a player from an adjacent court.

Three-Wall Strokes

Sidearm and Overhead Strokes

The nature of the three-wall game, with its higher bounces and lack of a back wall, forces players to develop the skill of using shots played chest high and above: the *sidearm* and *overhead strokes.*

The basic technique for the sidearm stroke utilizes all of the same principles of indoor strokes: backswing, forward stride, wrist snap, weight on the front foot, point of contact, maintaining eye focus, and follow-through.

The overhead motion is the same as in the four-wall game, but you should devote more time to developing this skill. Without a back wall to keep the ball in play, it becomes a higher percentage shot because it drives the ball into deep court.

Three-Wall Serves

While the basic service strokes and skills are the same for the three-wall game as for the four-wall game, the selection of angles often makes certain serves more effective. Instead of hitting a drive serve into the corners, *three-wall servers* may take a position at one end of the service zone and serve a drive serve at an extreme angle, so the ball lands inches past the short line and barely inside of the side line. This forces the receiver to pass the side line to return the serve; having to leave the confines of the court places the receiver in a poor position to return any ball hit to the opposite side of the court.

Another effective drive serve is when the server, while serving from the same end-of-service-zone position, uses a slightly wider angle, which results in the serve hitting deep on the side wall and barely crossing the short line as it caroms toward the center of the court. This serve is effective when it catches the receiver leaning or moving to the outside in anticipation of the serve leaving the court. Be warned, though: this can backfire if it's hit too deep or if it's anticipated, and may give the receiver an easy kill or passing shot.

A server taking this same position can also cross an opponent by utilizing a straight down-the-wall serve or sending a front wall–side wall serve to the side on which the server is standing. A hard drive serve can be effective when hit directly toward the receiver or slightly to the backhand side.

Another popular serve is a two-wall serve, similar to a "Z" serve in four-wall. Since there is no extended side wall, the serve is either hit chest-high and hard, ending up near the side line and forcing the receiver out of the court; or soft and high on the walls, landing near the rear line, forcing the opponent to return the ball on the fly or after bouncing deep in the court.

Another option is a wide angle, two-wall serve. This serve, which may be hit from either side of the service zone, makes contact with the front wall, high and near to the center. The ball then hits deeper on the side wall, near the service zone, keeping the opponent in deep court, returning serves from above chest-level.

Drive serve

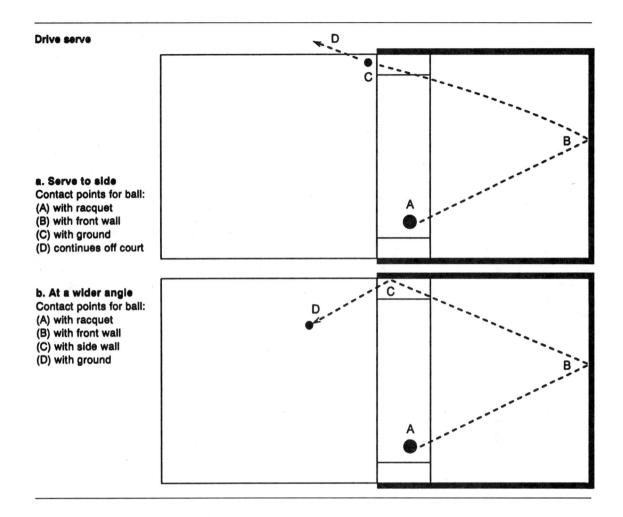

a. Serve to side
Contact points for ball:
(A) with racquet
(B) with front wall
(C) with ground
(D) continues off court

b. At a wider angle
Contact points for ball:
(A) with racquet
(B) with front wall
(C) with side wall
(D) with ground

Lob serves usually result in an on-the-fly return. If the receiver allows the ball to bounce, the result is often a difficult return from deep in the court, possibly past the end line. Lob serves may be ineffective, since most players attack the ball before the bounce and can end the rally with a good pass shot.

An overhand serve (one hit with a motion similar to throwing a baseball) is executed following a high bounce of the ball, and may result in a deep drive or a two-wall serve.

Basic serving strategy is to try to move the receiver near or past (outside of) the side line, leaving the entire court open for the next shot, or to keep the opponent deep in the court (near the rear line) for an easy drop shot. Once the server hits the ball a second time, the serving advantage is negated and neither player has an edge. Learn to serve effectively and to take advantage of this service edge to keep your opponent off balance. The goal of each serve should be to elicit a weak return from a player who is out of position.

Two-wall serve

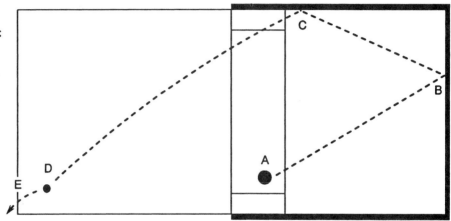

a. Basic serve
Contact points for ball:
(A) with racquet
(B) with front wall
(C) with side wall
(D) with ground
(D) continues off court

b. At wider angle
Contact points for ball:
(A) with racquet
(B) with front wall
(C) with side wall
(D) with ground
(E) continues past
    back line

Overhand serve

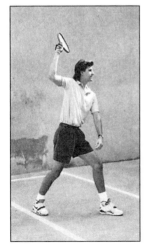 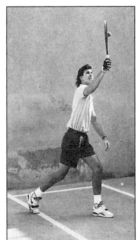 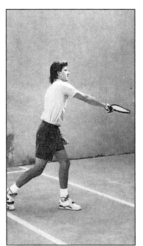 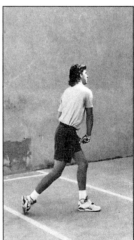

| a. Backswing | b. Contact | c. Swing | d. Follow-through |

Checklist for Three-Wall Serves

1. Service skills are mostly the same as in four-wall.
2. From one end of the service zone:
   ■ Use a wide-angle serve to force the receiver to make a return from past a side line.
   ■ Hit a serve that catches the last part of the side wall and rebounds just over the short line.
   ■ Hit a straight down-the-line drive serve.
3. A "Z" serve or wide-angle two-wall serve forces the receiver to return from outside of or deep in the court.
4. Lob serves may be dangerous because they usually elicit an on-the-fly return.
5. Basic serving strategy is to move the receiver to retrieve serves from outside of the side line or deep in the court.

Receiving the Serve

The *receiver* must be alert and ready to adapt to the large variety of serves that may be in the arsenal of the server.

Take a position in the center of the court, a few feet in front of the rear line. The depth will depend on the type of serves the server favors and the range and quickness of the receiver. The receiver should assume a stance with both knees slightly bent, weight forward on the toes, and racquet held high in the ready position. It is important that the ball be visually located as soon as possible in order to get a good jump on it.

The receiver must be able to move quickly to get into good body and racquet position for a solid return, especially when receiving a serve driven outside of the court. Use the basic principles of service return: make a crossover step, pivot and face the side wall (or the side wall extended), and position the racquet high to permit a smooth, full swing and follow-through.

Commonly chosen returns are the straight kill shot, pinch shot, down-the-wall pass, or "V" pass. A cross-court shot into the far corner will only come back to the server in the center court, giving him or her an easy shot.

The most difficult serve for most receivers to handle is the one that drives them past the side line and off of the court. The wall acts as a barrier for the ball and limits the surface available for the shot to hit. If the ball hits the outside of the wall on its way to the front wall, it results in a point for the server. This situation leaves only a part of the front wall or side wall as an available target.

If the receiver cannot bring about a side out with the service return shot, his or her objective should be to get a second shot and force a rally.

Checklist for Receiving Serves

1. Assume the ready position deep in the court and watch the ball as it is being dropped.
2. Popular returns are the straight kill shot, the pinch shot, down-the-wall pass, and the "V" pass.
3. Avoid returns that end up in center court.
4. If it is impossible to earn a side out, try to handle difficult serves with returns that will extend the rally.

The Rally

Once the rally begins and the players begin exchanging shots, the goal is to control the center area and keep your opponent to one side or deep in the court, which results in a lot of unreachable space for a well-placed shot to fall untouched.

When you force your opponent into making a long run off the court, he or she must stop and reverse momentum before changing directions and returning to the court. This is the time for you to make an easy drop shot or pinch shot to the opposite side of the court. This strategy can backfire, however, if the shooter tries to cut the shot too fine—instead of the ball landing close to the side line it lands over the line, resulting in an out and ending the rally.

The down-the-wall pass, the diagonal pass, or an out-the-door pass (one that forces the opponent "out the door" or off of the court) are very important skills to master in three-wall. These may be higher-percentage offensive shots than is the kill shot, because once they get past your opponent they are very difficult to return with good power.

Down-the-wall pass

Contact points for ball:
(A) with racquet
(B) with front wall
(C) continues off court

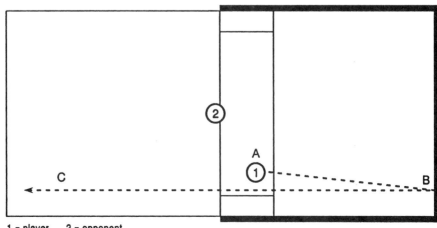

1 = player   2 = opponent

Out-the-door pass

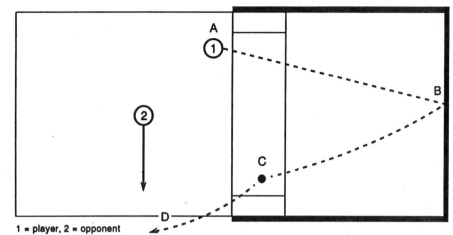

Contact points for ball:
(A) with racquet
(B) with front wall
(C) with ground
(E) continues off court: "out the door", with opponent in pursuit

1 = player, 2 = opponent

Out-the-door pass

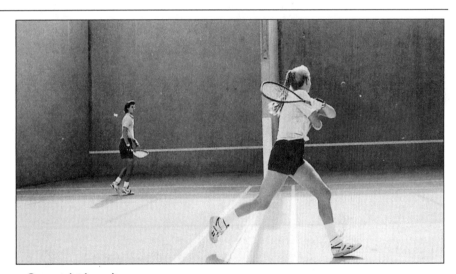

a. Correct (at knees)

✓	*Checklist for the Rally*

1. Try to gain control of center court.
2. Force your opponent to make long runs off of the court, "out the door" or near a side line, to return shots. This will leave you a lot of space that your opponent will find unreachable toward which to hit a rally-ending shot.
3. Be patient. Avoid hitting shots too close to the line, and wait until the opponent is out of position.

Summary

1. Three-wall facilities are found at many schools and parks and offer the opportunity to play the game of racquetball outdoors.

2. All the skills are the same as in four-wall, except the skills involving ceiling and backwall play.

3. In the absence of a back wall and deep side walls, shots must be played before they pass a player, thus making quickness and anticipation very important assets.

4. Rule differences are few, and mostly apply to the missing surfaces.

5. Court hinders that involve balls or players from adjoining courts are important safety considerations.

6. The main strategy of serves is to take advantage of the threat of being able to force a player to go outside of the court to retrieve a serve.

7. The receiver must be prepared to handle a variety of serves that require quickness and long runs to the ball.

8. Once driven outside of the court, a player must contend with a side wall, which blocks part of the ball's return path.

13   *Drills*

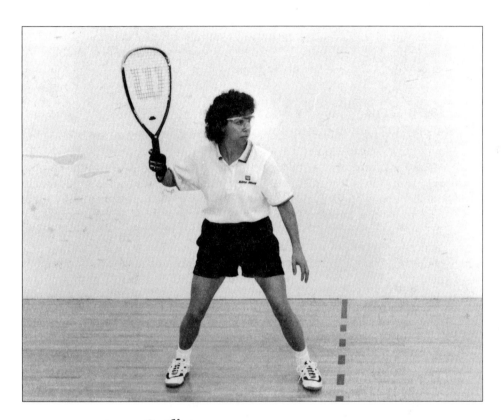

Outline

Introduction

The drills presented in this chapter can enable you to master the skills necessary to become an accomplished racquetball player. In order to learn the skills involved in any sport, an appreciable amount of time must be spent practicing them.

Drills are a means to this end. Drilling involves identifying the proper technique and repeating that technique until it becomes a learned movement—a habit. In order for a technique to become a habit, it must be repeated until correct execution feels natural and incorrect movements feel abnormal. Take the time to practice these drills until you have enough confidence in your ability to perform them during a fast-paced game.

Tape Drill

One drill intended to teach proper stroke technique requires a strip of masking *tape* and, if available, a partner.

Place the piece of masking tape on the floor somewhere deep in the back court area. The tape marks the spot on which to place the big toe of your back foot. If working on forehand strokes, the forehand side foot (right foot for right-handers, left foot for left-handers) will be on the line; for practicing backhand strokes, the non-racquet side foot (left foot for right-handers, right foot for left-handers) will remain on the tape. Do not move your foot from the mark. Remember from Chapter 3 that the rear foot will pivot but should not come off the floor.

Tape drill: Forehand   **Backhand**

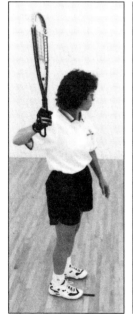 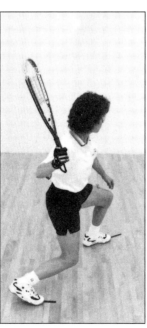 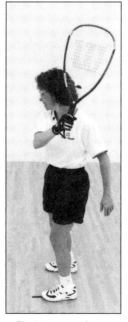 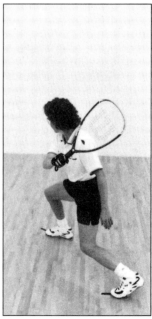

a. First tape mark   **b. Second tape mark**   **a. First tape mark**   **b. Second tape mark**

Checklist for Analyzing the Swing

On drills, check (or have a partner check) to see that you:
1. Are using a proper grip.
2. Bend at the knees (instead of the waist) to get down to the ball.
3. Swing flat.
4. Hit the ball when it is even with your forward foot.
5. Hit the ball when it is away from your body.
6. Follow-through fully.

From this position step out diagonally and take a series of full, healthy swings. Notice where your front foot lands after each swing (or have your partner note that spot). Freeze after each stroke and make adjustments to any incorrect technique, such as knee bend, hip direction, etc. When your forward foot consistently hits an area from where you can bend properly (bending from the legs, not the waist), mark that spot with another piece of tape.

The goal of this drill is to give the player a consistent distance for striding into the ball. This will allow for a smooth, consistent stroke each time.

Drop-and-Hit Drill

Using the same tape marks as in the first drill, *drop and hit* the ball. The tape is used to continue the consistency. Without the tape, most beginners tend to step at different angles and with different stride lengths, increasing the inconsistency of the shots.

Have a partner stand behind you, watching the swing and visually noting the relation of the stroke to your body. Your arm should move away from your body as it extends and moves through the ball. Have your partner mark with tape the center of the area the racquet passes over when your arm is fully extended.

With your feet positioned properly, drop the ball on the taped spot and swing through it. The ball should go straight to the wall and rebound straight back again, across that taped mark. If the trajectory of the ball is toward the near side wall, the ball is being hit too far back in the stance or too close to the body. Either situation will force the racquet face to open toward the side wall. If the ball rebounds across the court toward the wall behind your back, it was hit too soon—perhaps in front of the forward foot—or perhaps you snapped your wrist too quickly. Adjust this by dropping the ball a little behind the tape mark and see how the trajectory changes.

"Skip balls" hit the floor before they hit the front wall. This is probably the most frequent trajectory error and usually occurs from:

- Hitting too far behind the forward foot (hitting late)
- Hitting down, rather than flat, because of the pendulum action of the racquet (This often occurs because the player reaches down for the ball rather than bending at the knees for a level swing.)

Drop and hit drill

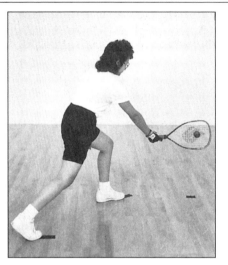 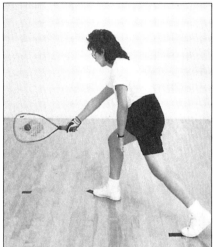

a. Forehand   **b. Backhand**

- The racquet face is down when the ball is being hit
- An incorrect grip, forcing the top edge of the racquet to be farther forward than the lower edge

Balls hitting too high on the front wall are another common problem. They are caused by:

- Hitting the ball too far in front of the forward foot (hitting early)
- Hitting up when making the upward pendulum swing of the racquet
- The racquet face being up when the ball is being hit
- An improper grip, forcing the bottom edge of the racquet head to be farther forward than the top edge
- Not bending at the knees

Continue with this drop and hit drill until the ball is going flat, hard, and straight, and the swing becomes automatic. When your form is perfect on this drill, move on to the next series of drills.

 Checklist for the Drop-and-Hit Drill

1. Take the proper grip.
2. Keep the toes of both feet on the foot portions of the tape.
3. Drop the ball on the ball portion of the tape.
4. Swing levelly.
5. Move the tape as needed to make any necessary corrections in the point of contact.

Footwork Drills

Step-Together-Step Drills

Beginning with a position near the back wall and facing a side wall, step sideways with the foot closest to the front wall. Slide the other foot up to that foot. Take another step with the foot closest to the front wall. Continue this shuffle step all the way to the front wall.

While still facing the same side wall, step with the foot closest to the back wall. Slide the other foot back. Step again toward the back wall. Continue this shuffle to the back wall.

Begin practicing these drills slowly, increasing speed as your skill improves. Repeat these shuffle drills until they feel comfortable, making certain that your feet never cross each other.

Step drill

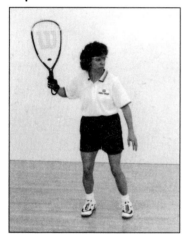

a. Feet together

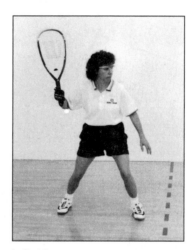

b. Stride

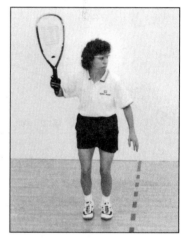

c. Feet together

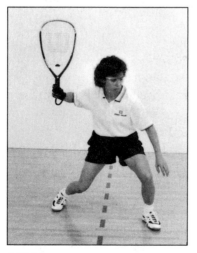

d. Stride

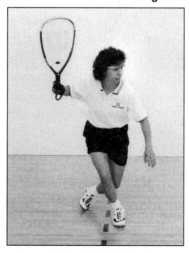

e. Do not allow feet to cross over

Star drill

From A to outlying numbers and back:

1. back-step, stride forward
2. step-together-step diagonally to and from
3. step-together-step to side and back
4. step-together-step diagonally to and from

5. stride forward, back-step
6. step-together-step diagonally to and from
7. step-together-step to side and back
8. step-together-step diagonally to and from

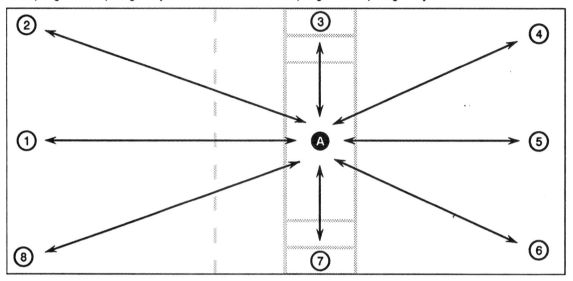

Star Drill

The star drill is a combination footwork and conditioning drill, in which the player covers the entire court in a star-shaped pattern as fast as possible while still maintaining proper footwork. Good technique is more important than speed in this drill. Do not sacrifice good form for speed.

- Start by facing the front wall in the center of the court.
- Back-pedal to point one.
- Run forward to the starting point.
- Step-together-step diagonally to point two.
- Step-together-step back to the starting point.
- While facing the side wall, step-together-step to point three.
- Step-together-step back to the starting point.
- Step-together-step to point four.
- Run forward to point five.
- Back-pedal to the starting point.
- Use the step-together-step technique to points six through eight.

Change Direction Drill

This two-person drill combines footwork and conditioning. A watch with a second hand is needed to time each sequence. The two participants alternate between running the drill and directing, which provides much-needed recovery time because of the strenuous nature of this drill.

The runner begins by facing the director and responds by moving in the direction indicated by the director's hand movements. If the director points at the runner, he or she responds by back-pedalling until the director points to signal a change in direction. A point away from the runner means a sprint forward. All hand movements to the side require the step-together-step technique.

This is an outstanding drill to teach quick direction changes and improve footwork speed.

Moving Ball Drills

Since you will have mastered the solid fundamentals of the preceding drills before trying the moving ball drills, your progress with these should be more rapid.

Side Wall Drill

Stand facing the side wall and toss the ball at it, letting the ball bounce once before hitting it. Get into hitting position as soon as the ball is released. Set up and hit straight at the front wall.

Footwork is crucial. One must be far enough away from the ball so that it is possible to take a full swing. There will be two movements:

1. Back and away from the ball, using step-together-step footwork
2. Striding into the ball, making sure there is enough room to extend your arm at the contact point (which is even with your front foot, at knee level)

Both of these motions can also be executed while taking diagonal steps backward. For the forehand, step back with the racquet-side foot, slide the other foot until both feet are together, then take another racquet-side step. This is a shuffle or step-together-step movement in which the feet do not cross each other. From this position, the next movement is to step forward with the non-racquet side foot, then swing forward.

Be certain that the movement of your body is away from the wall, so that the swing isn't crowded. Plenty of room is needed for a proper swing.

Front Wall Drill

Hit the ball toward the front wall. Hit it high and slow so that it takes time to get where it is going, giving you more time to adjust yourself to the return. The ball should bounce near mid-court. It is very important to concentrate on your footwork here, in order to get you to the point where you can hit the ball when it is at knee level or below. This generally requires that you move away from the ball. This takes discipline, because the natural instinct is to move toward the ball so that it can be hit quickly.

The first motion should be diagonally away from the ball. Do the step-together-step shuffle described above. Going straight back and then straight in will put the ball too close to the body. Move diagonally away from the ball toward a back corner. Then wait until the ball drops to about knee level, step into the ball, and swing levelly, hitting a low, straight shot at the front wall.

There are two other advantages to this footwork pattern. One is that with the hitter moving away from the ball, the opponent will have to commit to an area of the court. This allows the hitter to determine which shot will be the most effective. The other advantage is that by moving and being on his or her toes, the hitter can be active and assertive. The worst thing that a player can do is walk around the court, then plant the feet, and then hit the ball as it approaches, regardless of its height. The good player must strive for the best height on every shot.

By being active and alert you are ready for anything, mentally and physically. Alert play will make you more consistent. It will also unnerve your opponent, because you'll be more aggressive. In addition, it helps give you a much better workout!

Back Wall Drills

Most beginners and intermediates have trouble with balls coming off the back wall. Becoming proficient in the techniques of backwall play is a must for players at every level.

Barehand Drill

Put your racquet down, because it will not be needed for this drill. Stand about four feet from the back wall, with your racquet-side hand closest to the back wall. Face the side wall and toss the ball soft and high, so that it hits the back wall. As it bounces forward toward the front wall, move with the ball in the step-together-step shuffle. Each time the ball bounces, execute the shuffle step to get the feeling of moving with the ball.

Tossing the ball soft and high allows the player to move easily with the ball as it comes off the back wall. Keep the ball right in front of you as you both move toward the front wall. Alternate facing each side wall as you do this drill, so that you get practice moving with a forehand and a backhand shot.

The objective of this drill is to learn to coordinate body movement with the flow of the ball. On some of the bounces bend your knees more, as if hitting the ball at below-knee level for a kill shot.

This drill teaches timing and will point out flaws in improper footwork. An essential point in this drill is to be certain that the ball is in front of the body at the point of contact.

When you feel comfortable moving with the ball, the next step is to move with the ball until it has taken its first bounce off the floor. Let it bounce up, then, as it gets to knee level on the way down, catch it with your racquet hand. When you catch the ball, your hand should be in front of the forward foot, your arm extended away from the body—the position it should be in if you were hitting.

Players tend to get impatient and want to hit the ball while it is still high, rushing their shots. Practice letting the ball drop so that it is caught in front of the forward foot and below knee level. (This point cannot be emphasized enough.) Another tendency is to want to hit the ball before it has moved to a point in front of the forward foot.

A variation of this drill has the person being drilled freeze at the instant the ball is caught. The instructor or partner can check to see that the player's back foot has pivoted, the ball is below the knee and in front of the forward foot, the player's weight is forward, the knees are bent, and the body is not bent at the waist.

While beginners and intermediates can obviously profit from this drill, it is one that advanced players can also use when having problems with back wall shots. Remember, as with all drills, footwork, timing, and the point of impact are all essential.

Toss-and-Hit Drill

This drill is identical to the barehand drill, except that it is done with a racquet. The ball is tossed to the back wall, slow and high. The player does the step-together-step shuffle away from the wall, plants his or her rear foot, then hits the ball after its first bounce as it drops below the knee.

Simulated Game Drill

In this drill, the ball is hit hard to the front wall. As it bounces off the back wall, it is played before it takes its second bounce. Start by hitting easy, slow set ups. As your skill level increases, hit the ball to the back wall at different heights and speeds to give more variation and make the drill more gamelike.

Start by hitting straight down-the-line shots. After this skill becomes consistent, work first on cross-court and then pinch shots.

Ceiling Back Wall Drill

This drill allows you to work on taking a ball that has hit the ceiling, then the back wall (a common shot in racquetball).

A ceiling to back wall shot does not normally rebound very far from the back wall, so it is necessary to start nearer the back wall. But note that if the ball has been hit hard, it will rebound farther away from the wall. Once the ball rebounds from the back wall, start the step-together-step shuffle toward the ball.

There is a major difference between a ceiling ball coming off the back wall and a straight ball coming off the back wall. While the straight shot comes off straight, then gradually drops as it runs out of speed, the ceiling ball will drop quickly. Because it is dropping quickly, players often find themselves hitting the ball when it is behind them, or they are standing too straight and swing down at it. If the ball is traveling down and the racquet face is facing down on impact, a skip ball will be hit. Thus it is essential to make certain that the ball is in front of you when you hit it.

Keep your eyes on the ball the entire time. Watch it as it rebounds from the front wall, hits the back wall, then bounces. Taking your eyes off the ball, even for an instant, can reduce your chances of making an effective shot.

Ceiling Ball Drills

Solo Drill

In this drill, hit five consecutive forehand ceiling balls and then five consecutive backhand ceiling balls. These shots should hit the ceiling, but not the back wall or side wall. Don't ignore backhand ceiling balls, because in a game situation more ceiling shots are hit to the backhand side than to the forehand side.

On straight ceiling shots, the ball should be kept within five feet of the side wall. The next step is to hit cross-court ceiling balls from corner to corner. When you are successful with each shot five consecutive times, increase to ten.

Partner Drills

1. *Ceiling Ball/Conditioning Drill*

   After hitting the ceiling ball, run up to the center of the court. When the next ceiling ball is hit, run back and make the shot and then return to mid-court.

2. *Alternate Ceiling Balls*

   a. *Ceiling-Only Drill*   During a rally, return every ball to the ceiling unless it comes off a side wall or the back wall for a set up. This can be used strictly as a drill or it can be scored to add a greater element of competition. Here are some ways that it can be scored:

   - You score 1 point whenever the opponent hits a ceiling ball that hits the back wall or a side wall. Play to 11 or 15 points.

   - Play out every rally, allowing the opponent to go for the kill if a poor ceiling shot is hit. Play to 11 or 15 points.

   - Play out the rally, but even if the opponent just gets the racquet on the ball, he or she wins the point. This teaches the player to calculate the risk in hitting a low-percentage shot from the deep back court.

   b. *Corner to corner*   The two partners stand in the deep corners of the court, hitting ceiling balls to each other. One hits forehand and the other hits backhand. This lets one practice a backhand ceiling ball to the opponent's forehand, and the other practice a forehand ceiling ball to the opponent's backhand.

Service Drills

Serving Drills

Serving drills should be precise. It is not just getting the ball to the front wall and over the service line that counts; it is where the serve is directed that is important. By using tape to mark a target on the front wall, the server is forced to concentrate on perfection. Here are three drills to try.

1. Place a piece of tape on the front wall at the spot you think the ball should hit. The height will depend on the type of serve: drive, jam, etc. After each serve, make an adjustment to the tape, depending on where the serve lands. If a drive serve fails to cross the short service line, the target is too low. If you are attempting a down-the-line drive serve and it hits the side wall, adjust the angle by moving the tape to one side. Keep experimenting until you find the right target for each serve.

2. Place a target, such as a can of balls or a box, in a back corner of the court. Hit lob serves so that the ball hits the target just before it takes its second bounce.

3. Select one type of serve and see what percentage of serves hit or land near the target. Try to increase your percentage of perfect serves.

Serve-and-Return Drill

One player serves the whole 11-point game. The server wins a point if the receiver hits a weak return. The receiver gets a point if the return is a ceiling ball, passing shot, or kill. This is only a two-hit drill; each rally ends after the returner has hit the ball. Once the 11-point game is finished, the players switch positions and begin again.

Service Return Drill

Have a partner hit various serves. Practice different types of returns. For example, hit only ceiling balls for awhile, or have your partner hit serves off the back wall and practice passing shots or kills.

Summary

1. Drills are designed to help players of any level improve their form and technique.

2. Drilling without the ball can be valuable to learning the proper footwork.

3. The drop-and-hit drill is designed to improve stroke techniques.

4. The step-together-step or shuffle drill can help players learn to easily move forward and backward and get in position to execute a smooth, complete stroke.

5. Moving ball drills help a player learn to adjust to the different bounces the ball may take as it rebounds from the walls.

6. Specific drills are designed to assist players with whatever aspect of their game needs to be improved or made more consistent.

14 The Mental Side of Becoming a Better Player

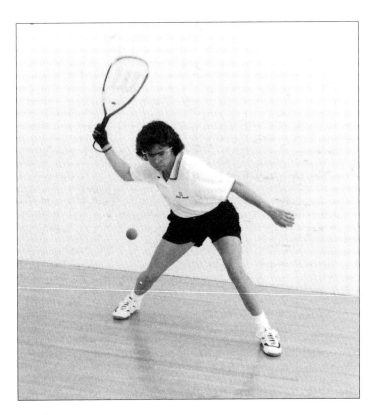

Outline

Wishing won't make you a better player. You must practice learning the physical skills of racquetball, and this practice can take place only on the court. It is also important to work out and condition your body. In addition, you can learn to become a better player off the court by practicing mentally. There are many skills to acquire in racquetball, and there are so many ways to practice that there should always be some way you can improve your game.

Mental Practice

Championship athletes have known for years that *mental practice* can help performance. Only recently have sport psychologists refined methods of utilizing the mind's contribution to the game.

Mental imagery, or *visualization,* is the name given to this type of mental practice. It can be done externally, by observing racquetball players or watching a videotape. It can also be done internally, by "feeling" yourself doing the action.

Another type of internal mental imagery involves you as the subject. You have only to close your eyes to see and feel yourself performing. (Golfer Jack Nicklaus calls this "going to the movies.")

While mentally experiencing your game, you can practice your strokes, footwork, or strategy. You can practice whatever aspect of your game you would like to improve. If your service return is a problem, imagine yourself ready for the return. Your imaginary opponent tosses the ball and hits to your backhand. Feel yourself stepping left with a crossover step, and starting your backswing, head down and eyes focused on the ball. You stride toward the ball and start your swing, following through and still focusing on the point of contact.

The following study serves to illustrate how mental imagery can help your game.[1]

Basketball players were divided into two groups. The first group physically practiced 100 free throws per day, while the second group was placed in a dark, quiet room and told to imagine that they were successfully shooting 100 free throws. In actual performance, the second group shot for a better percentage, because in their mental imagery they were successful on 100 percent of their shots, while the first group had missed some of the shots when practicing.

When using this technique with racquetball, imagine yourself doing everything correctly from start to finish (be sure to include a successful outcome!).

The following article demonstrates how mental imagery is a part of game preparation.

---

[1]Daniel Elon Smith, "Evaluation of an Imagery Training Program with Intercollegiate Basketball Players" (unpublished doctoral dissertation, University of Illinois at Champaign–Urbana, 1986), pp. 91–104.

Keeping Your Composure Through
Role-playing and Visualization[2]
by Lynn Adams

I frequently hear racquetball fans comment on the ability of the pros to consistently play well under pressure. How do they stay calm when most people would be nervous?

Well, there is no miracle answer, but there are ways to work to achieve that goal for yourself. One great difference between your type of practice and that of a pro's is that the pro's practice is geared specifically toward tournaments. Let's put physical skills aside and look more at the mental approach to the game.

Whatever your skill level, it would be reassuring to know that you could maintain that skill level consistently. But perfection, when you want it, is not guaranteed from any sort of drill or practice, although role-playing and visualization can help you calm down and play to your maximum skill level.

Let's talk about visualization first. Basically, players visualize their game and skill level in either a positive or negative manner. Many players are extremely hard on themselves. You see examples of this negative visualization when players yell at themselves or hit their racquets against the walls. These negative actions hurt a game more than help.

You need to work at developing a positive view of your game from the first day, an approach I've used to rise to win the Nationals this year. I have learned how to play whole matches in my mind before the game and I see myself hitting without hesitation, being quick, keeping calm and winning. But, believe me, learning this visualization skill has taken concentrated effort.

It all started one day when my coach, Jim Carson, asked me if I could see myself hitting a forehand. I tried it, and realized I couldn't. For a long time, I tried to imagine myself outside the court, looking in at myself. I tried to see myself the way others would see me, but I couldn't do it. I still can't. You never see yourself playing unless it's on video. That's why we're all so shocked to see ourselves on TV, because we never look the way we think we do.

Anyway, I gave up on that and tried visualizing myself on the court, feeling smooth, and seeing everything with the perception that I see when I'm actually playing. I could do that and found it really exciting. At that point, I started seeing myself hitting solid shots in the middle of my racquet. No matter what position I was in, I would hit my sweet spot.

You might want to start out by visualizing a drop and hit shot. Drop the ball and hit it straight, solid and low. Don't visualize a skip ball; be positive and hit a good kill or pass shot. If you have a problem seeing yourself doing this it may be because you haven't seen enough good players. You have to have some idea of what the shot should look like or feel

[2]Article reprinted from *National Racquetball,* August 1983, pp. 24–25.

like, so go and watch players with good, solid strokes. Looking at your stroke in a mirror also helps you form a picture in your mind of what you look like. Whatever your style, make your mental image positive.

After you can visualize a drop and hit, see yourself in a rally. See yourself up on your toes, ready to move quickly in any direction and in control of the situation. See yourself moving to the ball, setting up properly and taking a solid hit. You don't have to score right away. See yourself in long rallies, moving your opponent around, as well as in short quick rallies. A common problem among most players is nervousness or the lack of control over it. We get very emotional when competing and that creates all sorts of problems. If you want to see yourself in control of your own emotions, it must be done before you ever walk onto a court. You can't do it effectively in a pressurized situation. So, in your mind, put yourself at the start of a match and calm down, so that you're breathing normally, feeling good and your strokes are smooth. Put yourself in many situations and come out calm in all of them. Do this over and over until you can see and feel it clearly. Progress until you can play a whole match in your mind.

This gives you an idea of how to visualize. It takes time and practice, but it pays off. Like any other drill you do, if you cheat or rush through this exercise, it will do you no good at all.

Role-playing goes hand-in-hand with visualization and you add the dimension of writing to it. We (Jim and I) do a lot of role-playing and it helps me a lot. Role-playing is planning ahead for what might happen. I put myself into different situations and think of as many different possibilities to that situation as I can. Then I figure out how I would want to react to each possibility. For instance, I'm in a close tie-breaker, and my opponent goes for a shot and gets it on two bounces. She doesn't call it and neither does the ref. I lose the rally and the appeal. Since line judges are split in what they saw, she gets the point. In my mind, I know she cheated. That's my situation. Now I go through the possible reactions.

First, I get very angry and confront her. She just smiles and turns away, which heightens my anger. Knowing how I react, if I get too upset, I will dump the next shot and lose another point. That's definitely not a good solution.

Next, I could ignore it, figuring it's part of the game and out of my control and go on to play the next point. I could calmly express to my opponent that it's too bad her confidence in winning is so low that cheating is necessary to score points. That's usually a good way to make my opponent feel guilty. If the crowd saw her cheat, I could get them in on making her feel badly. I could yell at the ref for making a lousy call, etc.

There are always options available. By thinking of them in advance, I choose how I react. That doesn't mean I'm always in control of every situation, because I'm definitely human, but I am in control most of the time.

In case you're wondering which option I would have chosen in the given example, if I were in total control of myself, I would say the line about not having confidence. But that's effective only if I can say it without hostility and if I truly feel sorry that my opponent had to stoop to that level.

Otherwise, I'd ignore it and concentrate on the next rally. I want to do what's necessary for me to score that next point.

Another form of role-playing is to place yourself in specific situations. It's 10–10 in the tie-breaker and I have a ceiling ball that comes up short and I have the opportunity to shoot the ball. What shot do I hit? Be sure to thoroughly define the situation. Where is my opponent? How fast is she? Who has the momentum? Whose serve is it? How have I been hitting the last four or five shots?

By playing these pressure points in advance, over and over in different ways, they are a little less scary when they actually happen. If you wait until it's actually 10–10 before you ever think about what shot you should hit, you'll tense up and miss whatever you try. Think about it in advance.

I role-play all sorts of things, on and off the court. Something I think is important is being a gracious loser as well as winner. You can throw your tantrums when you're alone, but not in front of a crowd. So, I role-play losing a match I wanted to win very much and practice controlling my temper. I'll role-play a victory speech so I don't forget to thank someone who is important, and I role-play a game in front of a crowd that wants me to lose. There are so many situations that come up in competition, and the more prepared you are, the better you'll handle yourself.

Where does the writing come in? I write a lot of this down on cards and take them to my matches. I'll write down my game plans (played out in advance), write down my opponent's strengths and weaknesses, write down my playing goals, i.e., always be aggressive, hit through the ball, tentativeness will make you lose a point, etc. I also write down tendencies of mine when I let the pressure get to me. That way I can go to my cards and let them remind me of things, because when I start losing it in a match, I forget lots of things, and having thoughts written down in advance helps me focus and calm down. It helps me concentrate on positive things instead of getting upset about losing a game, a point or my cool. Also, writing helps me pull all my thoughts together. It makes me concentrate on racquetball and what I'm trying to accomplish and tune out everything else. That in itself is a fantastic role-play for a match. When you're playing a match, you want to be able to tune out all distractions and focus on playing the ball. I think one of my strong points is being able to concentrate totally for long periods of time. I can tune out a whole crowd; comments an opponent may make, etc., to the point where I actually don't hear them. I'll hear a general murmur-type noise, but it's quiet, and I can't hear specific words. I know I'm able to do that, because visualization and role-playing take a lot of concentration. When you get to the point where you can concentrate long enough to visually see yourself play a whole game, you're well on your way to being able to do that in an actual tournament.

To me, the real joy of playing racquetball comes when you get past the physical aspect of the game. When I'm able to take my physical game and

Checklist for Mental Imagery

1. Watch top-level racquetball players or videotapes of racquetball skills.
2. Be the star in your own "movie" by closing your eyes and performing racquetball skills to perfection.
3. When using mental imagery, always see yourself completing all aspects of the skill perfectly, including a successful finish.
4. Practice all aspects of the game mentally.

make it better by using my head, that excites and inspires me to get even better. I realize that it's hard to concentrate on anything else when your main concern is just getting the ball to the front wall, but these techniques are to be used before you walk onto the court. If you feel you're not ready to do these types of things yet, that's fine. Whenever you try it, do it with energy and do it for a while. Don't try it once, get frustrated and quit. The mind side of the game takes practice just like your forehand or serve. It's no different, and patience will reward you.

Relaxation

Relaxation is another essential to playing good racquetball. Practice taking a slow, deep breath before preparing to serve. This can help clear your mind so you can concentrate on the serve. It can also help you relax your muscles between periods of action. If your muscles are relaxed, you are more prepared for the smooth, effortless stroke necessary in the sport of racquetball. Tense muscles tend to inhibit smooth, efficient activities and speed up the onset of fatigue.

To teach yourself to get the most out of relaxation and deep breathing, sit quietly in a chair with your eyes closed and concentrate on slowly taking and releasing deep breaths. You can say to yourself "breathe in, breathe out," or repeat a nonsense syllable such as "om" or "one." Concentrating on this syllable repetition is designed to help you relax by eliminating all tension-causing thoughts from your mind. By emptying your mind as you concentrate on your breathing, your muscles will relax and your blood pressure can be lowered. If other thoughts come into your mind, return to your breathing pattern and verbal repetition. This is the basis for many of the benefits that can be gained from the practice of meditation.

After you have learned to relax while sitting calmly in a quiet place, the next step is to transfer that ability to the racquetball court.

Checklist for Learning to Relax

1. Sit, completely relaxed, on a comfortable chair in a quiet room.
2. Close your eyes.
3. Slowly take in and release a deep breath while repeating a meaningless syllable; this repetition should help you to relax by blocking all tension-causing thoughts from your mind.
4. If other thoughts come into your mind, don't worry. Just get back into your breathing pattern and your syllable repetition.

Concentration

Concentration is the third major area of mental practice. The most important object on which to concentrate in racquetball is the ball. Failure to focus on the ball from the serve and through the point of contact (which includes the point at which the ball is on your racquet) is probably the most common and critical error at every level of racquetball. Slow-motion studies reveal that most people take their eyes off of the ball when it is still four to six feet away from them. They look at the target point on the wall instead of concentrating on the point of contact of the ball and racquet. A good way to combat the tendency to look up at the last moment is to remember the phrase, "Keep your eyes on the ball, instead of the wall."

Concentrate on seeing the ball as it comes off of the wall, while it is on your racquet, and continue to focus on the point of contact even after the ball has left your racquet. Keeping your eyes focused on the point of contact prevents you from lifting your head, shoulder, and hips and allows you to maintain a level swing to complete your follow-through.

 Checklist for Concentration

1. On the court, the most important object to concentrate on is the ball.
2. Focus on the ball from the first possible moment until after the ball has left your racquet.
3. "Keep your eyes on the ball, instead of the wall."

Goal Setting

Another important aspect of the mental side of the sport is setting both long-term and short-term *goals.* (Short-term goals assist in achieving long-term goals.)

After you decide on your long-term goals, make plans to achieve them. An example of a long-term goal is a desire to be the champion of the semester-ending class tournament.

Short-term goals involve improving the specific skill or skills necessary to achieve your long-term goal. Examples of short-term goals are improving your drive serve to the backhand corner, learning to wait longer on kill shots, or improving your ceiling shots.

Once you've set a goal, develop a practice schedule designed to increase your chances of attaining it. If you want to increase your ability to play a back-hand shot off the back wall, you can engage in mental practice along with your on-court repetition. Visualize different shots, some low, some high, bouncing toward or away from your position.

With visual practice, you can start your physical practice. Hit yourself some balls that come off the back wall. Have a partner feed you some similar balls. Analyze what you have done right and wrong on your practice shots.

Summary

1. In addition to practicing physical drills, the complete racquetball player must make maximum use of his or her mental faculties if serious about improving his or her game.

2. Mental preparation includes:
   - *Imagery,* in which a person visualizes the techniques and game situations that he or she may encounter
   - *Relaxation,* in which a player can avoid tension and perform to a higher level
   - *Concentration,* in which the player focuses on the ball all the way to the point of contact

3. Goal setting is important for all areas of our lives. If effectively applied to racquetball, it can speed up both skills improvement and enjoyment of the game.

15 *Fitness for Racquetball*

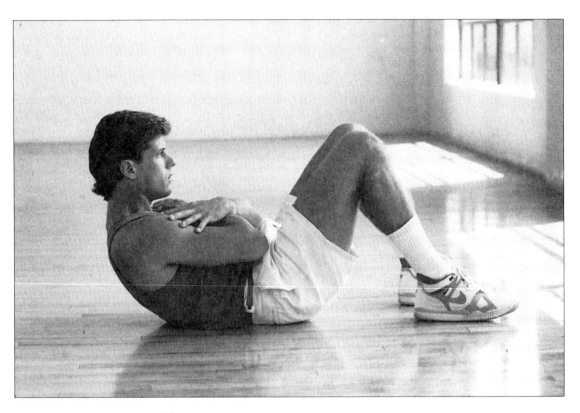

Outline

Proper execution (bouncing on the toes, raising the arm high on the backswing, pivoting on the shot, getting into good position, and maintaining concentration) is mandatory for playing winning racquetball. However, *fatigue* is a primary limiting factor to proper execution.

How many times have you heard the statements "I blew so many easy shots" or "I cramped up"? These excuses can often be attributed to fatigue. Injuries, too, are often the direct result of fatigue (e.g., pulled muscles, strains, sprains, and muscle soreness). As players get tired they make more errors and stumble, leading to injury. Being in shape for racquetball can aid in avoiding these pitfalls and help one to increase enjoyment in playing the game.

Of course, a person can just go onto the court and play an easy game of tapping the ball to the front wall, but if you want to get into the spirit of the game and be able to maintain a high level of skill throughout the match—*get into shape!*

Training is specific—the only way to get into shape for racquetball is to play racquetball. Although running, basketball, cycling, lifting weights, etc., will not condition you to play racquetball, they can condition your body to be more receptive to the racquetball training regimen and to have reserve power when it is needed.

The first step to improved fitness is to increase the capacity of your cardiovascular system (heart, lungs, and arteries), enabling it to supply oxygen to all of the muscles in your body for a period of time long enough to maintain the pace of an extended rally or an all-day tournament.

Strong muscles are a great help when that extra step, snap, rotation, or support is needed. Specific strength-building exercises can also help prepare the body to withstand the strain of competition with less chance of injury.

Flexibility is also desirable, so you can execute the quick body twists and all-out reaches without injuring muscles or placing excess strain on joints.

Overload Principle

The main factor in improving fitness of any kind is the *overload principle.* *Overload* means that during each workout you should do a little more than you are accustomed to doing. If you never overload, you'll never see improvement.

There are three ways to overload:

- *Intensity*—How hard you do something
- *Duration*—How long you do something
- *Frequency*—How often you do something

Intensity may be measured by monitoring your pulse rate, either during or immediately following exercise. The higher your pulse rate, the harder your heart is working. A task should become easier to perform as your condition improves, thus enabling you to work at higher intensities (all-out play for a longer period of time). Intensity means playing at an elevated degree of speed, power, and concentration: all-out play, going full blast for every point, pressing your opponent, cutting down rest time between serves, etc.

Duration is measured by how long a period of time you continue to exercise. Playing for longer periods each time you play will gradually condition your heart to be able to work longer and longer without rest.

Frequency is measured by how often you play. As your condition improves, so will the amount of time you can spend on court.

In order to improve your cardiovascular system, you must overload one or more of these areas of fitness. The area that it is safest and easiest for the body to overload is frequency. This may be accomplished by playing more times per week at the same intensity.

Aerobic Training

You can improve your cardiovascular system by performing exercises that elevate your pulse rate for an extended period of time. These activities, known as *aerobic exercises,* increase the body's ability to supply oxygen to its cells.

In order to contract, muscle cells need fuel, which they receive from blood cells in the form of nutrients. The nutrients are metabolized from the food we eat. Oxygen is necessary in order for the cells to utilize these nutrients. When the heart and lungs cannot supply oxygen at a rate fast enough to keep up with the demands placed on it by the body (a phenomenon known as *oxygen debt*), fatigue sets in and efficiency decreases.

Aerobic exercises train, or condition, the body to adapt to this demand by strengthening the mechanisms involved: the heart, lungs, and arteries. Dr. Kenneth Cooper is the person responsible for making *aerobic,* an obscure physiological term that literally means "with oxygen," a household word. He defined aerobics as a variety of activities that stimulate heart and lung activity for a time period sufficiently long to produce beneficial changes in the body. Dr. Cooper calls these changes a *training effect.*

A training effect increases the efficiency of the lungs (allowing them to process more air with less effort), increases the efficiency of the heart (allowing it to pump more blood with each stroke), increases the number and size of the small blood vessels (capillaries), increases total blood volume, and improves the tone of your muscles and blood vessels.

The bottom line is that exercising aerobically increases maximal oxygen consumption by improving the efficiency of the supply and delivery of oxygen to the body's cells. You may select any activity that keeps your pulse rate in the target pulse zone (discussed in the next section) for an extended period of time. The most commonly recommended activities are running, jogging, cycling, stationary running, rope jumping, walking, and swimming.

Aerobic activities are those that elevate the pulse rate to a level high enough to attain a training effect, but not so high as to cause fatigue or the need for rest. The individual should be able to continue the exercise for a length of time long enough to attain a training effect. Experts differ on the exact minimum length of time, but it ranges from 12 to 30 minutes per training session. The intensity level for such activities should be low, the duration of the activity should be long, and breathing should remain fairly regular.

Checklist for Benefits of an Aerobic Training Effect

1. *Increases efficiency of the lungs*—Enables them to process more air with less effort.
2. *Increases efficiency of the heart*—Increases its stroke volume, enabling it to pump more blood with each stroke.
3. *Increases the number and size of blood vessels*—The arteries become stronger and the capillaries increase in number.
4. *Increases total blood volume*—The body produces more blood cells to meet greater demands.
5. *Improves muscle tone*—The muscles become fitter and the muscle layer of the arteries becomes stronger.
6. *Changes fat weight to lean weight*—Increases the lean body mass (percentage of muscle in the body).
7. *Increases maximal oxygen consumption*—Improves the efficiency of the supply and delivery of oxygen to the body's cells.

Target Pulse Zone

One way to ensure that you are exercising aerobically is to monitor your pulse rate to keep it in the *target pulse zone*—the pulse level that the body should maintain in order to reap the benefits of aerobic training. To learn your target pulse zone, you must first determine your maximum exercise pulse, which is found by subtracting your age from 220. Your target pulse zone is between 65 and 80 percent of your maximum exercise pulse. If an activity is too intense for you, your pulse will rise above the upper limit of your target pulse zone, and your breathing will become more difficult as a result of your body's attempt to keep up with this extreme oxygen demand.

Example: $\begin{array}{r} 220 \\ \underline{- \text{ 20 years old}} \end{array}$

$200 \times 80\% \ (.8) = 160$
$200 \times 65\% \ (.65) = 130$
Target Pulse Zone is between 130 and 160 beats per minute

This individual should maintain a pulse rate inside of these parameters for his or her body to receive the benefits of aerobic training.

The key to being able to receive maximum benefits from aerobic activities is to exercise longer, not harder; low-intensity, long-lasting, continuous aerobic training periods help your body become able to continue performing for longer periods of time and to delay the onset of oxygen debt and fatigue while playing racquetball.

Taking pulse rate

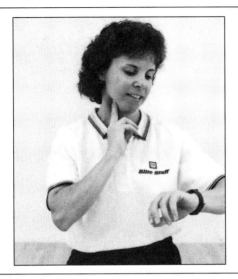

Anaerobic Exercise

Another type of exercise demands oxygen at a rate faster than the body can provide—*anaerobic exercises. Anaerobic* literally means "without oxygen." Such activities are so intense that they cannot be maintained for a long period of time. Exercises or sports involving stop-and-go activity, such as racquetball, tennis, basketball, and soccer, are usually considered anaerobic instead of aerobic activities because they are so intense and have periods of inactivity.

Other examples of anaerobic activities are 100-yard dashes, weight lifting, and continuous fast-breaks in basketball. After engaging in such activities for only a short time the individual must stop and rest, usually panting to allow the body to replenish its oxygen stores. During anaerobic activities the pulse may be extremely elevated and breathing irregular (panting).

✓ Checklist for Comparing Aerobics and Anaerobics

Characteristics	
Aerobics	Anaerobics
Low intensity	High intensity
High duration	Low duration
Pulse slightly elevated	Pulse highly elevated
Continuous, uninterrupted regular breathing	interrupted by rests, Irregular breathing (panting)
No oxygen debt	Oxygen debt; fatigue;
Burns fat as fuel	Burns carbohydrate as fuel

Anaerobic Training

Racquetball often has periods of very intense activity, so the body must be conditioned for them. This may be attained by playing harder—more intensely for longer periods of time, resulting in an overload.

Other activities that may increase the body's ability to maintain a high intensity level are those that bring the pulse rate above the target pulse zone. Examples of this type of activity are running sprints, bicycle sprinting, running up long flights of stairs, and continuous jumping.

Summary

1. Proper conditioning can allow a player to maintain a high skill level throughout an entire game and avoid fatigue-induced errors and injuries.
2. Training is specific. In order to get into shape to play racquetball, you must play racquetball.
3. Racquetball conditioning demands improvement of the cardiovascular system, strengthening of the muscles, and increased flexibility of the joints.
4. For best results, the overload principle should be the basis for your fitness program.
5. There are three ways to overload: intensity, duration, and frequency.
6. Aerobic training can improve the efficiency of the cardiovascular system.
7. Aerobic training results in the phenomenon known as a *training effect*.
8. Anaerobic exercises are activities of higher intensity and lower duration, while aerobic exercises are activities of lower intensity and higher duration.
9. In order to benefit from aerobic activity, your pulse rate must remain in the target pulse zone all during the activity.
10. Since racquetball is primarily an anaerobic activity, improved fitness may be gained through playing racquetball at a more intense level for longer periods of time and by activities that duplicate these high-intensity demands, such as sprinting, climbing, and other explosive activities.

16   *Gaining Strength and Flexibility and Avoiding Injuries*

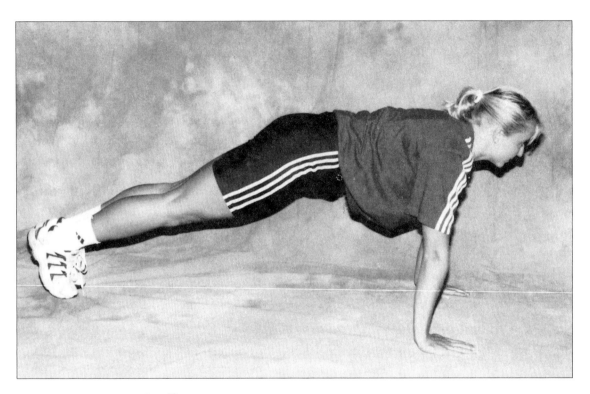

Outline

I t was only a few years ago that strength training for athletes was taboo; now it is a necessity. The idea that working with weights made people muscle-bound has given way to the truism that strength and flexibility training are essential for every athlete. Shot putters and discus throwers were the first to use resistance training. Then came football players. Soon all athletes found that strength training could greatly increase their abilities. As a racquetball player, you too can profit from strengthening your body.

Strength

Strength is essential for most athletic events. In racquetball, leg strength is needed to move and to make every shot. Abdominal and shoulder strength are essential to move through the ball smoothly and effortlessly. And wrist strength is necessary for every shot. Maximum strength is gained by exhausting your muscles in a few repetitions.

Wrist strength, actually forearm strength, is essential. About half of beginners don't have the necessary strength to swing the racket up and hammer the ball down toward the court. Also, many players get "tennis elbow" as a result of weak forearm muscles and tendons. To gain wrist strength you should do wrist curls with weights. A simple way to gain forearm strength quickly is to simply hold the end of a broom, palm down, then raise the broom. This will strengthen the muscles needed for your backhand. For your forehand do the same exercise with the palm up.

Wrist Curls

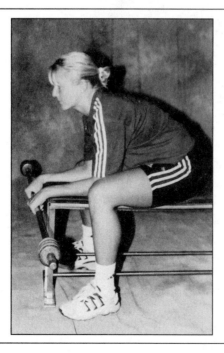

Broom Curl for forearm strength

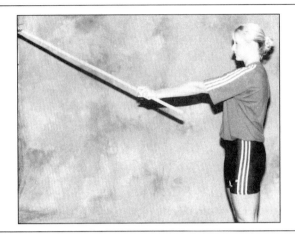

Manual resistance for forearm strength

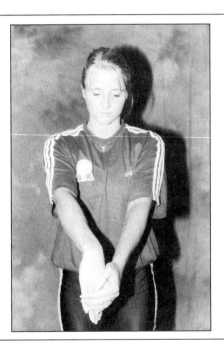

The exercise can also be done using manual resistance. For the backhand put finger pressure on the back of one hand and extend the wrist. This can be done on the palm of the hand for forehand strength or on the back of the hand for backhand strength. Bring the bent wrist through 180 degrees.

Squeezing a ball or a grip strengthener are great for stronger hands and forearms.

Triceps strength is needed for the backhand. The triceps are weak in most people, so additional strength can help you to bring the racket through quickly.

Pushups for tricep strength

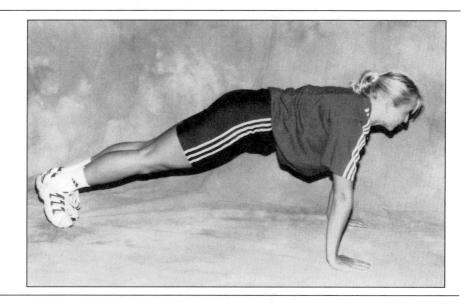

Strengthening upper back muscles

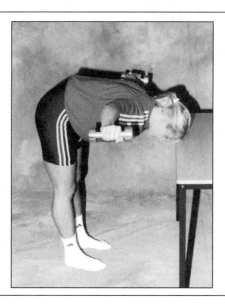

A push-up will help to gain strength for the triceps in the backhand and for the upper chest for the forehand.

To develop triceps strength with manual resistance. Bend your right arm by touching your shoulder with your hand. Now take the other hand and place it against the wrist of your bent arm. Straighten your arm as you give yourself resistance.

Upper back muscles are used in hitting the backhand. If you have dumbbells, take one in each hand, bend over, and lift the dumbbells up to your side.

Leg extensions

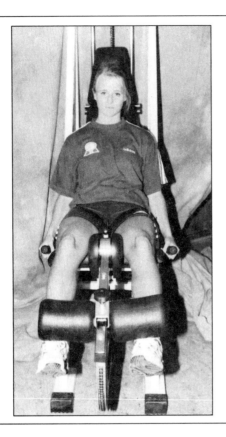

Leg power can be developed by simply jumping. Or if you have access to weights or a gym, do leg extensions, presses, or half-squats.

Back extensions are done on a Roman Chair. Bend forward, then raise straight back. This exercise can also be done on the floor. Lie on the floor face down and, arching up just a little, slightly lift your shoulders and knees just off the floor. Don't lift your chest and knees more than two inches off the floor. (If you arch up too high it is called a "hyperextension," and this is not a recommended exercise.) These lower back muscles are often injured in everyday activities, so this exercise should be done throughout your life.

Abdominal muscles are best strengthened with abdominal curl-ups. With your knees bent and your back on the floor, curl forward, keeping your hips (belt) on the ground. This is another good lifelong exercise.

The inner and outer parts of your hips can be strengthened on a special hip machine, if one is available, or on a pulley. For hip flexion, have the pressure on the front of the leg and bring the leg forward. For hip extension, which is the primary running action, have the pressure on the back of the leg or ankle and bring the leg backward. For the outside of the hips, which are used in quickly stepping sideways, have the pressure on the outside of the leg and move the leg outward. The inside of the hip is also important because it is also

Back arch

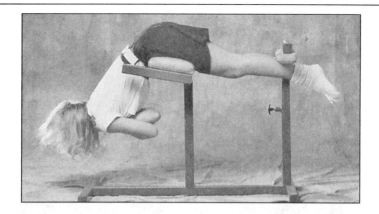

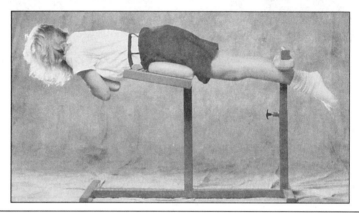

Abdominal curl-up

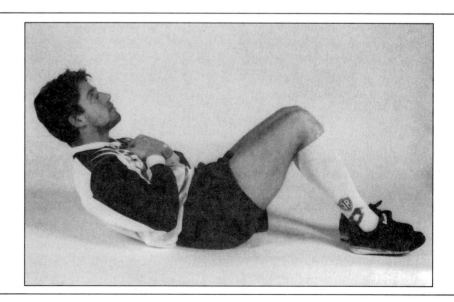

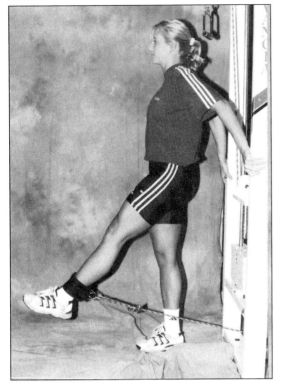

Hip flexion

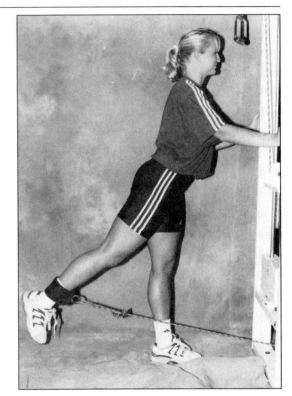

Hip Extension

used in sideways movement. Starting with the leg outward and the pressure on the inside of the leg, bring the leg inward. You can also do these exercises with a partner giving you the resistance. Lie on your back with your legs in the air, and have your partner grasp your ankles. Push your legs out with the partner resisting. Then pull your legs in with your partner again resisting.

Flexibility and Warm Up

You need good flexibility throughout your body in order to move smoothly through a full range of motion in every stroke and serve. These flexibility exercises may be done after you have completed your playing. While we have traditionally done stretching as a part of the warm up, this practice is now being questioned by sport researchers. Studies with runners have found that those who warmed up by stretching have more injuries than those who don't. No studies have been done on racket sport players as yet.

Another negative of prepractice stretching is that it reduces what is called "muscle stiffness." When muscle stiffness is reduced it reduces one's power. Studies with weight lifters and swimmers have shown a reduction in power after stretching in a warm up.

Strengthen sideways motion

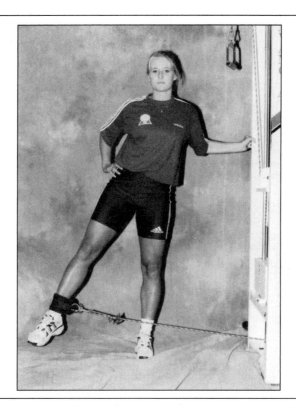

Strengthen sideways motion

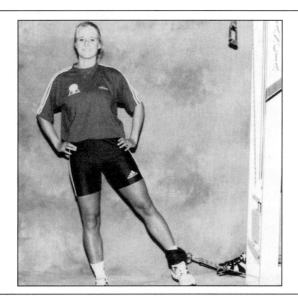

Stretch upper chest

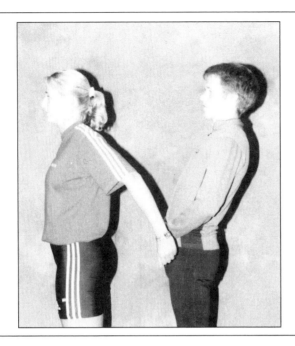

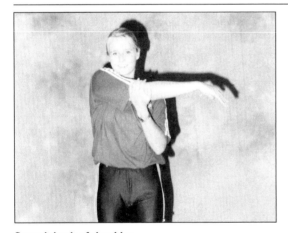

Stretch back of shoulder

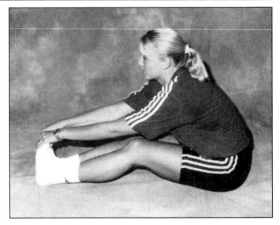

Stretch Hamstrings

Gaining flexibility is different from warming up. If your arms or legs will not go through a full range of movement sufficient for you to play the game effectively, you will need some extra flexibility. Flexibility is better gained after the muscles are warmed up. If you need more flexibility, for example in your calf muscle, stretch after practice and stretch farther, holding the stretches longer. Stretching when you are very warm is more likely to result in greater permanent flexibility. Hold each stretch for 20 to 30 seconds.

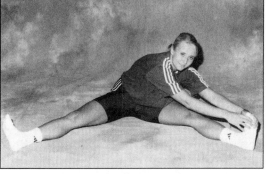

Stretch Groin

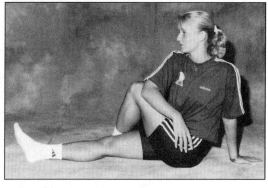

Abdominal stretch for flexibility

The upper chest is stretched by bringing your arms to shoulder level, then pulling them backward as far as they will go. For the upper back, bring them forward as far as possible and cross them. You can also have a partner pull back on your arms to stretch the connective tissues in the front of your shoulders.

To stretch the back of the shoulder, which may be needed if your backhand backswing is restricted, pull your arm across your chest and hold.

For the rear of the thighs, while sitting slowly bend forward and touch your toes. If it is done standing, be sure to bend your knees slightly.

Groin area muscles are stretched by spreading your feet about three feet, bending your legs, then moving your torso over one leg, then the other.

Calf muscles are stretched by standing with your toes on a raised board, then letting the heels lower to the floor. It can also be done by standing three or four feet from a wall or fence and leaning on the support. With your legs straight and heels on the ground, drop your hips lower until you feel the stretch.

Flexibility in the abdominals is gained by placing one foot on the outside of the opposite thigh, then twisting the torso away from that foot.

Aerobic (Cardiopulmonary) Conditioning

To develop your heart's ability to deliver oxygen to your muscles, you need to get your heart beating fast for a long time. Six minutes is an absolute minimum to make any improvement, and for proper conditioning you should work for at least 20 to 30 minutes with your heart rate at the target level.

The traditional method of determining your target heart rate is to merely subtract your age from the number 220, then work out with your pulse rate at a level of 65 to 90 percent of that number. Suppose you are 20 years old: 220 minus 20 equals 200, and a target rate of 65 percent would be 130 heart beats per minute, while a target rate of 85 percent would be 170 beats per minute. (See Box for Karvonen's more complicated, and more commonly accepted, method.)

Karvonen's Formula for Determining your Target Heart Rate

Scientists are continuing to improve their knowledge of how best our bodies can work. The Finnish scientist Karvonen has improved on the simple formula of 220 minus your age as the maximum heart rate. He starts with that number but then subtracts the resting pulse rate to determine the "heart rate reserve."

1. First take 220 minus your age _____ . This is your maximum heart rate (MHR).
   Next you will need to determine your resting pulse rate. Take this while lying in bed in the morning before you get up. Use your index and middle fingers and locate your pulse either on the side of your neck (carotid artery) or on the wrist just above the thumb. Count the number of pulse beats in a minute or take your pulse for 15 seconds and multiply by 4 to determine the total for a minute.

2. Resting pulse rate (Rest HR) _____

3. Subtract the resting pulse rate from the maximum pulse rate.
   Answer for first of the above questions minus the answer for the second.
   MHR _____ − Rest HR _____ = _____ heart rate reserve (HRR)
   Now you will determine your maximum and minimum pulse rates for an effective work out. For the average person your high end will be your heart rate reserve multiplied by 80% (.80) then add to that number your resting pulse rate.

4. _____ (HRR) × .80 = _____ + _____ (Rest HR) = _____ Maximum desirable heart rate during exercise.
   Next find the minimal acceptable level for your work out by taking the heart rate reserve (HRR), multiplying it by 60% (.60), then adding in your resting pulse rate.

5. _____ (HRR) × .60 = _____ + _____ (Rest HR) = _____ Minimal desirable heart rate during exercise.
   These two percentages (60% and 80%) are not set in stone. If you had medical problems or were in very poor condition you might use a number between 40% and 55% to set your minimal pulse rate. If you were very fit or a competitive athlete you might use 85% or 90% to set your high-end exercise pulse rate.
   An example of how a 20-year-old would determine the target training pulse range. Assume that her resting pulse rate was 70.
   Minimum target heart rate (220 − 20 = 200 + 70 = 270) × .60 = 162
   Maximum target heart rate (220 − 20 = 200 + 70 = 270) × .80 = 216
   For a 40-year-old with a resting pulse of 65 the target heart rates would be:
   Minimum target heart rate (220 − 40 = 180 + 65 = 245) × .60 = 147
   Maximum target heart rate (220 − 40 = 180 + 65 = 245) × .80 = 196

Checklist for Preventing Blisters

1. File down any calluses so that blisters do not develop under them.
2. Always wear socks when you are wearing shoes.
3. Use two pair of socks, especially early in the sport season.
4. Buy shoes with a proper fit and break in new shoes gradually.

Any manner in which you can reach that level is acceptable. You can run, skip rope, cycle, or play continuous racquetball (in which you keep running—you run while you rally, you run to pick up a ball, and you run back to your position). You can also condition yourself aerobically by playing imaginary racquetball. Play against an imaginary partner with no ball. Practice your footwork and your shots.

Common Injuries and How to Avoid Them

The facts that racquetball is generally played on a hard surface, hitting a ball which is often going quite fast, with a racquet extending the arm and transferring significant force to the elbow and shoulder give racquetball some potential for injury—although they are nowhere near as common as injuries from playing tennis. The most common injuries are called "overuse" injuries because they occur over time after weeks, months, or years of strains on the muscles, tendons, and bones.

The chronically stressed elbow can have muscular, tendon, or bursa damage and is seen in "tennis elbow," in another type of tendinosis such as "little league elbow," or in a softened or damaged cartilage (chondromalacia). The third type of injury can be a rupture of one of the elbow ligaments in a single overhead smashing movement.

Tennis elbow (lateral humeral epicondylitis) can affect anyone who has continued strain on the back of the forearm. It is most common on the outside of the arm just under the elbow. It is caused primarily by hitting backhand shots. The muscles in the back of the forearm are not as strong as those on the inner side of the forearm, so they are more likely to be injured. This type of tennis elbow is most frequently found in recreational players.

You can also have a tennis elbow problem on the inside of the elbow. This is most likely caused by hitting hard forehand drives and overheads, but the continued hard forehand drives also contribute to the problem. The problem of tennis elbow on the inside (medial) part of the elbow is more common among elite players. This type of tennis elbow (medial epicondylitis) is also found in other athletes and may be called "golfer's elbow" or "pitcher's elbow" depending on the sport. It is an inflammation of the tendons on the inside of the elbow—caused by the straightening (extending) of the arm.

Elbow problems occur in some people. They are only 33 percent of those found in tennis players. Vibrations from the racquet are a primary cause of the repeated stress to the forearm muscles and the elbow. When the ball is hit, the farther from the middle of the racquet (the sweet spot) that you hit the ball, the more vibrations are developed. So the beginner is much more likely to incur elbow problems. Their muscles are not conditioned to the sport and their coordination is not good enough yet to hit the ball in the middle of the racquet on every stroke.

What to do:

1. RICE (Rest, ice, compression, elevation).
2. Wear an elbow brace specifically designed for the condition. Most sporting goods stores and tennis shops stock them.
3. To prevent a recurrence, or to prevent it from happening in the first place, do wrist extension exercises. A reduced-vibration racquet, such as the titanium racquet, may help.

Prevention of tendon and muscle problems in the elbow can be done if the muscles around the elbow are strengthened so that they absorb more of the shock of the force. For example, to prevent a tennis elbow one should do reverse wrist curls or, more simply, just grasp the end of a broom and, with your palm facing down, lift the broom using only the movement of the wrist. Do this several times each day to strengthen the muscles on the back side of the forearm. This strengthens the arm for backhand drives. To prevent the tennis elbow problems that occur on the inside of the forearm, lift the same broom with the palm of the hand facing upward. Use only wrist movement.

Chronic low back pain is a common complaint of more skilled players. Tight buttock and hamstring muscles, tight connective tissue in the lower back, poor abdominal strength, poor posture (sway back), and muscle strains are the most common.

Knee pain can affect every aspect of the knee. Pain in the front of the knee ("housemaid's knee," prepatellar bursitis) can be caused by a number of injuries, including damage to the patellar tendon or an inflamed bursa (lubricating sac). It can be caused by continued trauma to the area or by a weakness of the hamstrings when compared with the quadriceps, which puts additional pressure on the front of the knee.

Damage to the back surface of the knee cap (patella) is medically termed *chondromalachia patella* (injury to the back of the knee cap) or *patelliofemoral pain syndrome* but is commonly called "cyclist's knee" or "runner's knee." There are many causes, including the misalignment of the knee cap caused by a lack of flexibility, muscular weakness in the quadriceps, by a bone deformity, or by a roughening of the smooth cartilage lining of the patella, which doesn't allow it to ride smoothly in its most desired track.

Patellar tendonitis is common at all ages among runners, jumpers ("jumper's knee"), and with some racket sport players. The continued flexion and extension of the knee joint during running can cause minute damages to the tendon. In more severe cases the tendon can tear in the area of the patella or closer to the tendon's attachment below the knee.

Blisters are caused by an irritation of the skin in which the skin is rubbed and the outer layer of skin separates from the inner layer. When too much friction is put on the skin, it heats the skin and acts like a burn. This causes a blister. The first and second layers separate and the fluid from the second layer fills that separation. The more friction and the more heat produced, the larger the blister. The fluid inside the blister causes pain.

They are most common on the back of the heel, on the toes, or under the ball of the foot. Stiff-heeled shoes, shoes not properly laced, shoes that are too big or too small, and new tennis shoes are often the cause of a blister. At the beginning of a sport season blisters are far more likely. It is always a good idea to wear two pair of thin socks when breaking in new shoes. The extra sock absorbs some of the rubbing that the skin would otherwise have to endure. If you notice a special pressure when you are active, paint the area that feels irritated with tincture of benzoine ("Tuff Skin") and then cover that with a cream or gel such as Vasoline.

What to do:

1. Use a donut-shaped pad around the blister to eliminate any more pressure.
2. Use a skin lubricant, such as Vasoline, over the blister to protect from any additional stress.
3. Keep the area clean because the blister may pop on its own and you do not want to invite infection.

To prevent blisters:

Plantar fasciitis is a common complaint, especially with older athletes. It is said to affect nearly 20% of runners. The soreness is under the foot and in the heel or just forward of the heel. "Plantar" means the bottom of the foot, "fascia" is the connective tissue (tendons and ligaments), and "itis" means inflammation. It is usually caused by bruising the tissue on or near the heel.

Plantar fasciitis may occur in several tissues in the bottom of the foot. The most common area is on or just in front of the heel bone (calcaneus). The ligaments and tendons that attach to the heel are prone to problems from either trauma, overstretching, or tightening due to not being stretched often enough. Tight calf muscles and tendons (gastrocnemius and soleus) are often related to the cause, so stretching of the heel is always recommended as part of the cure. Stretching of the rear calf muscles should be done several times a day. The muscles that move the bones of the foot may also be bruised or stretched.

Another related cause is often that the foot is pronated (the inside part of the foot is closer to the ground). When this is true a proper orthotic device, which lifts the long arch of the foot, may both heal the foot and prevent a recurrence. The orthotic may take up to six months to cure the problem.

The pain is particularly noticeable when getting out of bed in the morning. It may also be evident when arising after being seated for some time. The condition is generally a stress injury in which the tendons under the foot are repeatedly stressed, as in running in tennis. Rest is the major type of treatment. A doughnut pad or a rubber heel cup with extra cushioning underneath may also be an aid. Arch supports, which are made for increasing the arch of the foot, can also help.

Arch problems affect many people. There are two arches in the foot. One is under the base of the toes (the transverse arch) and the other runs from the front of the heel to the base of the toes (the metatarsal arch). These arches act as shock absorbers. Extra high or very low arches sometimes cause problems. An orthotic that is inserted under a low arch will bring the foot closer to normal and will generally relieve any pain.

Very high arches may also cause problems, but an orthotic can give support. If the high arch is caused by tight connective tissue (ligaments and tendons) under the foot, hammer toes or plantar fasciitis may result.

Orthotics are shoe inserts that generally affect the heel and both arches of the foot. Properly designed, they reduce both foot, ankle, and lower leg problems. They are valuable in preventing or healing plantar fasciitis, shin splints, fallen or weak arches, and a number of other problems. Racquetball players have found them to be helpful in holding the foot in its proper position and in making their shoes fit more effectively. Medical doctors, podiatrists, and chiropractors can all fit you for orthotics. There are also some orthotics that you can purchase from sporting goods stores and which may work for you. They are made for the traditional problems in feet and may or may not work perfectly for you.

Heel cups can reduce or prevent some problems. The hard plastic heel cups can make up for poor-fitting heels in your shoes. The soft rubber heel cups can absorb shocks and help to prevent or ease those problems in which continued stresses occur. Heel spurs, plantar fasciitis, and shin splints can be aided by rubber heel cups.

Summary

1. The complete racquetball player must make use of his or her maximum mental and physical potentials. There are proven ways to improve one's tennis off the court.
2. Physical conditioning requires that the racquetball player develop strength, flexibility if needed, and cardiovascular endurance.
3. For a racquetball player, strength and flexibility are most important in the thighs, groin, upper chest, back, triceps, forearms, and abdominals.
4. Proper conditioning and equipment can reduce the chance of injury.

17 *Nutrition for Better Health*

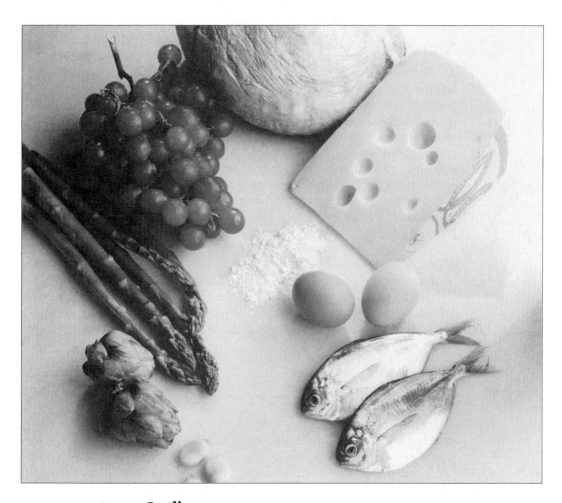

Outline

A long and full life requires exercise, an adequate diet, and play—both physical and mental—and a basic understanding of the science of nutrition is essential to healthy living. If you are going to play soccer you will need adequate fuel for your athletic body. This chapter describes the basic elements of good nutrition. In the next chapter we will discuss how to apply these nutritional principles to your diet and weight management.

Nutrition

An informed person is aware of the nutrients necessary for minimal function, and can then put that knowledge into practice by developing a proper diet. Unfortunately, very few people consume even the minimum amounts of each of the necessary nutrients—protein, fat, carbohydrates, vitamins, minerals, and water (the essential nonnutrient). The first three nutrients listed (protein, fat, and carbohydrates) provide the energy required to keep us alive, in addition to making other specific contributions to our bodies.

The calorie measure used in counting food energy is really a kilocalorie—one thousand times larger than the calorie used as a measurement of heat in your chemistry class. In one food calorie (kilocalorie), there is enough energy to heat one kilogram of water one degree Celsius, or to lift 3,000 pounds of weight one foot high. So those little calories you see listed on cookie packages pack a lot of energy.

Most people need about 10 calories per pound of body weight just to stay alive. If you plan to do something other than just lie in bed all day, you probably need about 17 calories per pound of body weight per day in order to keep yourself going. And if you play a good deal of soccer, you can count on using a whole lot more calories.

Protein

Protein is made up of 22 *amino acids,* which consist of carbon, hydrogen, oxygen, and nitrogen. While both fats and carbohydrates contain the first three elements, nitrogen is found only in protein. Protein is essential for building nearly every part of the body—the brain, heart, organs, skin, muscles, and even the blood.

There are four calories in one gram of protein. Adults require 0.75 grams of protein per kilogram of body weight per day; this translates into one-third a gram of protein per pound. So an easy way to estimate your protein requirements in grams per day would be to divide your body weight by three. For instance, if you weigh 150 pounds, you need about 50 grams of protein per day.

Physically active adults have been thought to require more protein than is recommended by the United States Recommended Daily Allowance (USRDA), which is set at .8 grams per kilogram of body weight per day. In fact, most active people do not need to eat additional protein if 12 to 15 percent of their total calories is protein. Since active individuals need to consume more calories per day than their inactive counterparts due to their increased energy expenditure, active adults who keep their protein intake at around 15 percent of their total calories will eat more protein per day and thereby fulfill their body's protein requirement. Excess protein consumption (above the body's requirement) is broken down and the calories are either burned off or stored as fat.

However, when you are involved in a strenuous strength training regimen, as you might be if you play competitive golf, it may be necessary to increase your protein intake percentage, depending on the number of total calories you consume per day.

In order for your body to make any kind of tissue, including muscle, you must first have all of the necessary amino acids. Your body can manufacture some of them, while you must get others from your food. Those amino acids that you must get from your food are called the *essential amino acids,* while the others that you can make are known as the *nonessential amino acids.* During childhood, nine of the 22 amino acids are essential, while in adulthood we acquire the ability to synthesize one additional amino acid, leaving us with eight essential amino acids.

Amino acids cannot be stored in the body, so we need to consume our minimum amounts of protein every day. If adequate protein is not consumed, the body immediately begins to break down tissue (usually beginning with muscle tissue) to release the essential amino acids. If even one essential amino acid is lacking, the other essential ones are not able to work to their capacities. For example, if methionine (the most commonly lacking amino acid) is present at 60 percent of the minimum requirement, the other seven essential amino acids are limited to near 60 percent of their potential. When they are not used, amino acids are excreted in the urine.

Animal products (fish, poultry, and beef) and animal byproducts (milk, eggs, and cheese) are rich in readily usable protein. This means that when you eat animal products or by-products, the protein you consume can be converted into protein in your body because these sources have all of the essential amino acids in them. These foods are called *complete protein sources.*

Incomplete protein sources are any other food sources that provide protein but not all of the essential amino acids. Examples of incomplete proteins include peas and nuts. These food sources must be combined with other food sources that have the missing essential amino acids so that you can make protein in your body. Examples of complementary food combinations are rice and beans or peanut butter on whole wheat bread.

Another reason to be aware of complementary food combinations is that they enhance the absorption of the protein consumed. The person who is aware of the varying qualities of proteins can combine them to take advantage of the strengths of each. For example, if you eat flour at breakfast in the form of a piece of toast or coffee cake and wash it down with coffee, then drank a glass of milk at lunch, each of the protein sources would be absorbed by your body at a lower level. But if you ate bread with the milk at either meal, the higher protein values of both would be absorbed by your body immediately.

Fats

Fat is made of carbon, hydrogen, and oxygen. There are nine calories in a gram of fat. In the body, fat is used to develop the myelin sheath that surrounds the nerves. It also aids in the absorption of vitamins A, D, E, and K, which are the fat-soluble vitamins. It serves as a protective layer around our vital organs, and it is a great insulator against the cold. It is also a great concentrated energy source. And of course its most redeeming quality is that it adds flavor and juiciness to food!

Just as protein is broken down into different kinds of nitrogen compounds called amino acids, there are also different kinds of fats. There are three major kinds of fats, or fatty acids: saturated fats, monounsaturated fats, and polyunsaturated fats.

Saturated fats are "saturated" with hydrogen atoms. They are generally solid at room temperature and are most often found in animal fats, eggs, and whole milk products. Since these are the fats that are primarily responsible for raising the blood cholesterol level and hardening the arteries, they should be minimized in your diet.

Monounsaturated fats (oleic fatty acids) have room for two hydrogen ions to double-bond to one carbon. They are liquid at room temperature and are found in great amounts in olive, peanut, and canola (rapeseed) oils. Dietary monounsaturated fats have been shown to help the body excrete dietary cholesterol, thereby contributing a positive effect on atherosclerosis, one type of arteriosclerosis.

Polyunsaturated fats (linoleic fatty acids) have at least two carbon double bonds available, which translates into space for at least four hydrogen ions. Polyunsaturated fats are also liquid at room temperature and are found in the highest proportions in vegetable sources. Safflower, corn, and linseed oils are good sources of this type of fat. Polyunsaturated fatty acids of the omega-3 type may also contribute to the prevention of atherosclerosis.

We eat too much fat. The minimum requirement for fat in the diet is considered to be somewhere between 10 and 20 percent of the total calories consumed. The absolute maximum should be 30 percent, which is the amount now recommended for the American diet. While we as a society are still above this 30 percent value, we have been declining since the 1970s, and we need to keep that trend going. Most of us consume between 35 and 50 percent of our total calories in fats, with a very high percentage in saturated fats—the fats that we want to avoid.

Our high fat intake, most of which is saturated, tends to raise blood cholesterol levels in many people. If you are interested in decreasing the chances of developing hardened arteries by lowering your blood cholesterol level, it is recommended that you follow a diet low in fat (with the saturated fat intake at 10 percent or less of your total diet) and consume less than 300 milligrams of cholesterol daily. Or to put it another way, keep the total calories from fat under a third of your total intake and eat twice as much polyunsaturated and monounsaturated fat as saturated fat.

In the past, companies were allowed to identify the oil in a product on their labels as simply vegetable oil; under the Food and Drug Administration requirements made in 1976, they are now required to note whether it is corn oil, cottonseed oil, soybean oil, and so on, because some oils, even though they are not of animal origin, are very high in saturated fat. Palm kernel oil and coconut oil, often referred to as "tropical oils," are particularly high in saturated fats.

When you buy foods, especially cookies and crackers, always check the type of fat used. Avoid those with palm kernel oil and coconut oil. Also be aware of the hydrogenated oils used. While a hydrogenated safflower or canola oil may still have an acceptable fat ratio, a hydrogenated peanut or cottonseed oil may not contain the desired levels of unsaturated fats. Partially hydrogenated vegetable oils may contribute to the development of heart disease. The dietary use of hydrogenated corn oil stick margarine has been shown to increase LDL cholesterol levels when compared to the use of similar amounts of corn oil, also indicating an increased risk of heart disease.

In terms of controlling one's blood cholesterol level, dietary cholesterol is not as important as saturated fats in your diet. For this reason, saturated fats such as red meats, butter, egg yolks, chicken skin, and other animal fats should be greatly decreased. As an informed consumer, you may want to keep track of both your total fat intake and your intake of saturated fat to become better aware of your potential risk for heart disease. For example, one egg contains 5.6 grams of fat and only 0.7 grams of polyunsaturated fat, while an equal weight of hamburger contains 8.7 grams of fat and only 0.4 grams of polyunsaturated fats.

Carbohydrates

Carbohydrates are made from carbon, hydrogen, and oxygen, just as are fats, but "carbs" are generally a simpler type of molecule. There are four calories in a gram of carbohydrate. If carbohydrates are not utilized as immediately for energy as sugar (glucose), they are either stored in the body as glycogen (the stored form of glucose) or synthesized into fat and stored. Some carbohydrates cannot be broken down by the body's digestive processes; these are called fibers and will be discussed later. Digestible carbohydrates, can be separated into two categories: simple and complex. *Simple carbohydrates* are the most readily usable energy source in the body and include such things as sugar, honey, and fruit. *Complex carbohydrates* are the starches, which also break down into sugar for energy, but their breakdown is slower than with simple "carbs." Complex carbohydrates also bring with them various vitamins and minerals.

People in the United States often eat too many simple carbohydrates. These are often referred to as "empty calories," because they have no vitamins, minerals, or fibers. While a person who uses a great deal of energy can consume these empty calories without potential weight gain, most of us find these empty calories settling on our hips. The average person consumes 125 pounds of sugar per year, which is equivalent to one teaspoon every 40 minutes, night and day. Since each teaspoon of sugar contains 17 calories, this amounts to 231,000 calories or 66 pounds of potential body fat if this energy is not used as fuel for daily living.

High-carbohydrate diets that are especially high in sugar may be hazardous to one's health. They can increase the amount of triglycerides produced in the liver. These triglycerides are blood fats and are possible developers of hardened arteries. Also, a diet high in simple carbohydrates can lead to obesity, which can then result in the development of late-onset diabetes.

Fiber

Fiber is that part of the foods we take in that is not digestible. Fiber helps to move food through the intestines by increasing their peristaltic action. Vegetable fibers are made up chiefly of cellulose, an indigestible carbohydrate that is the main ingredient in the cell walls of plants. Plant-eating animals, such as cows, can digest cellulose. Meat-eating animals, such as humans, do not have the proper enzymes in their digestive tracts to metabolize cellulose.

Bran—the husks of wheat, oats, rice, rye, and corn—is another type of fiber. Bran is indigestible because of the silica in the outer husks. Some fibers, such as wheat bran, are also insoluble. The major function of fiber is to add bulk to the feces and to speed digested foods through the intestines. This reduces one's risk of constipation, intestinal cancer, appendicitis, and diverticulosis.

Some types of fibers are soluble; that is, they can find and eliminate certain substances such as dietary cholesterol. Pectin, commonly found in raw fruits (especially apple skins), oat and rice brans, and some gums from the seeds and stems of tropical plants (such as guar and xanthin) are examples of soluble fibers that pick up cholesterols as they move through the intestines.

Foods high in fiber are also valuable in weight-reducing diets because when foods pass more quickly through the digestive tract, the time available for absorption is reduced. Fiber also cuts the amount of hunger experienced by a dieter because it fills the stomach. A large salad with a diet dressing might give you very few calories, but it contains enough cellulose to fill your stomach, cut hunger, and move other foods through the intestinal passage.

Food processing often removes natural fiber from our food, and this is one of the primary reasons that we in the western world have relatively low amounts of fiber in our diet. For instance, white bread has only a trace of fiber—about nine grams in a loaf—while old-fashioned whole wheat bread has 70 grams. And when you peel a carrot or an apple, you remove much of the fiber.

Dietitians urge us to include more fiber in our diets. People should be particularly conscious of the benefits of whole-grain cereals, bran, and fibrous vegetables. Root vegetables (carrots, beets, and turnips) and leafy vegetables are very good sources of fiber. The average American diet has between 10 and 20 grams of fiber in it per day. This low level of fiber is believed to account for the fact that we have about twice the rate of colon cancer as do other countries whose citizens eat more fiber. This is why the National Cancer Institute has recommended that we consume between 25 and 35 grams of fiber per day.

Checklist for Effective Eating

1. Eat 12 to 15 percent of your diet in proteins, preferably fish, fowl without skin, and beans.
2. Keep your fat intake between 10 and 30 percent of your total calorie intake, with saturated fat intake 10 percent or less and a higher proportion of monounsaturated fat.
3. Most of your diet should be complex carbohydrates (less-refined products) such as whole wheat, fruits, and vegetables.
4. It is recommended that people supplement with antioxidant vitamins (beta carotene, vitamins C and E).

Vitamins

Vitamins are organic compounds that are essential in small amounts for the growth and development of animals and humans. They act as enzymes (catalysts) that facilitate many of the body's processes. Although there is controversy about the effects of consuming excess vitamins, nutritionists agree that we need a minimum amount of vitamins for proper functioning.

Some vitamins are soluble only in water; others need fat to be absorbed by the body. The water-soluble vitamins, B complex and C, are more fragile than the fat-soluble vitamins, because they are more easily destroyed by the heat of cooking, and if they are boiled, they lose some of their potency into the water. Since they are not stored by the body, they should be included in the daily diet. However, even though they are not stored in the body, it is still possible to ingest too many water-soluble vitamins, leading to kidney stones because of the excess demand placed on the kidneys for processing.

The fat-soluble vitamins, A, D, E, and K, need oils in the intestines to be absorbed by the body. They are more stable than the water-soluble vitamins and are not destroyed by normal cooking methods. Because they are stored in the body, there is the possibility of ingesting too much of them—especially vitamins A and D.

Although nutritional researchers disagree about whether vitamin supplements are necessary, many of them see the necessity for supplementation with the vitamins that neutralize free oxygen radicals. Free oxygen radicals are harmful substances produced by many natural body processes, air pollution, and smoke, and seem to be responsible for some cancers and other diseases. Physical exercise, for all of its benefits, is one producer of free oxygen radicals.

Supplementation with antioxidants (beta carotene, vitamins C and E) reduces free oxygen radicals in the body. Dr. Ken Cooper, the man who coined the term "aerobics" and developed the first world-recognized fitness program, suggests a minimum supplementation of 400 IU of vitamin E, 1,000 mg of vitamin C, and 25,000 of beta carotene daily to counteract the potential damage done to the body by free oxygen radicals.

Minerals

Minerals are usually structural components of the body, but they sometimes participate in certain body processes. The body uses many minerals: phosphorus, calcium, and magnesium for strong teeth and bones; zinc for growth; chromium for carbohydrate metabolism; and copper and iron for hemoglobin production in the blood.

Iron is used primarily in developing hemoglobin, which carries oxygen in red blood cells. Women need more iron (18 milligrams a day) than men until they go through menopause, at which time their iron requirements drop to that of men (10 milligrams a day). Iron deficiency, common in women athletes, may impair athletic performance and should be corrected with supplementation.

Magnesium is the eighth most abundant element on the earth's surface. It seems to help activate enzymes essential to energy transfer. It is crucial for effective contraction of the muscles. Exercise depletes this element, so supplementation may be called for. When it is not present in sufficient amounts, twitching, tremors, and undue anxiety may develop.

Calcium is primarily responsible for building strong bones and teeth. For this reason, it seems obvious that a diet that is chronically low in calcium would have a negative effect on one's bone strength. Low calcium intake results in brittle and porous bones as one gets older, a condition known as osteoporosis. This is diagnosed when bone density shows a loss of 40 percent of the necessary calcium. It happens quite often in older people, especially women who have gone through menopause or have had their ovaries removed, because estrogen seems to protect against bone loss.

In teenage and young adult years, the inclusion of adequate calcium (which may be higher than the current Recommended Daily Allowance, or RDA) can aid in the development of peak bone mass, which can help prevent osteoporosis later on in life. Another contributing factor to osteoporosis is the imbalance of phosphorus to calcium in the typical diet. Calcium and phosphorous work together, and should be consumed on a one-to-one ratio. However, the average diet is much higher in phosphorus than calcium, leading to a leaching of calcium from the bones to make up for this imbalance.

Calcium is also necessary for strong teeth, nerve transmissions, blood clotting, and muscle contractions. Without enough calcium, muscle cramps often result. Skipping milk with its necessary calcium may be the cause of menstrual cramping for some girls. The uterus is a muscle, and muscles need both sodium and calcium for proper contractile functioning.

Phytochemicals

Phytochemicals (phyto is the Greek word for "plant") include thousands of chemical compounds that are found in plants. Some of these are vitamins and many have no known effect on us; however, more and more are being found to be highly beneficial.

In the past, the phytonutrients found in fruits and vegetables were classified as vitamins: Flavonoids were known as vitamin P, cabbage factors (glucosinolates and indoles) were called vitamin U, and ubiquinone was vitamin Q. Tocopherol somehow stayed on the list as vitamin E. The vitamin designation was dropped for other nutrients because specific deficiency symptoms could not be established. "Vita" means "life," so if the compound could not be found to be absolutely essential for life, it was dropped as a "vitamin," but is now classified as a phytochemical.

Various phytochemicals have been found to reduce the chance of cancers developing, reduce the chance of heart attack, reduce blood pressure, and increase immunity factors. Few of these have been reduced to pill form, such as vitamin pills, so they must be consumed in fruits and vegetables daily. It is suggested that each of us consume at least five servings of raw fruits or vegetables daily. Since many of the phytochemicals are heat sensitive, cooking can destroy some or all of the active ingredients.

We are a long way from developing highly effective phytochemical supplements, because there are so many elements and they may be destroyed in the processing. Garlic pills, for example, are available. However, in the deodorized versions, some active ingredients have been removed—they were in the chemicals that give garlic its "aroma."

Several types of phytochemicals are being studied. *Plant sterols* are somewhat similar to the animal sterol cholesterol but are unsaturated. These plant sterols compete for the same sites and thereby lower the blood cholesterol levels by as much as 10 percent. Soy is a good source for such sterols. Most green and yellow vegetables, and particularly their seeds, contain essential sterols.

Phenols have the ability to block specific enzymes that cause inflammation. They also modify the prostaglandin pathways and thereby protect blood platelets from clumping, thereby reducing the risk of blood clots. Blue, blue-red, and violet colorations seen in berries, grapes, and purple eggplant are due to their phenolic content.

Flavonoids is the name for a large group of compounds found primarily in tea, citrus fruits, onions, soy, and wine. Some can be irritating, but others seem to reduce heart attack risk. For example, the phenolic substances in red wine inhibit oxidation of human LDL cholesterol. The biologic activities of flavonoids include action against allergies, inflammation, free radicals, liver toxins, blood clotting, ulcers, viruses, and tumors.

Terpenes such as those found in green foods, soy products, and grains comprise one of the largest classes of phytonutrients. The most intensely studied terpenes are carotenoids—as evidenced by the many recent studies on beta carotene. Only a few of the carotenoids have the antioxidant properties of beta carotene. These substances are found in bright yellow, orange, and red plant pigments found in vegetables such as tomatoes, parsley, oranges, pink grapefruit, and spinach.

Limonoids are a subclass of terpenes found in citrus fruit peels. They appear to protect lung tissue and aid in detoxifying harmful chemicals in the liver.

Recent research confirms suspicion of the effects of soy products and related foods, which have long been used in Oriental diets. It has long been observed that Oriental women do not experience the problems of menopause, such as hot flashes, that western women commonly endure, but until recently, no theories have been advanced. Now we realize that a major factor is the fact that the Asians eat more vegetables, particularly soybeans.

It is phytoestrogens—plant chemicals that mimic the effects of the female hormone estrogen—that seem to be the major factor. These plant-like estrogens have similar effects to the natural estrogen in reducing heart disease, maintaining brain functions, reducing the incidence of breast cancer, and reducing softening of the bones (osteoporosis). In addition, other positive effects, which may or may not be related to estrogen intake, also occur, such as reduction in cancers (prostate, endometrial, bowel) and the effects of alcohol abuse[1].

Water

Water is called the essential nonnutrient because it has no nutritional value, yet without it we would die. Water makes up approximately 60 percent of the adult body, while an infant's body is nearly 80 percent water. Water cools the body through perspiration, carries nutrients to and waste products from the cells, helps cushion our vital organs, and is an essential element of all body fluids.

The body has about 18 square feet of skin that contains about 2 million sweat glands. On a comfortable day, a person perspires about a half-pint of water. Somebody exercising on a severely hot day may lose as much as seven quarts of water. If this is not replaced, severe dehydration can result. It is therefore generally recommended that we daily drink eight 8-ounce glasses of water or the equivalent in other fluids. This amount is dependent on the climate in which you live, the altitude at which you live, the type of foods that you eat, and the amount of activity that you participate in on a day-to-day basis. Golf can be strenuous and makes us sweat—**so** be sure to drink plenty of water when you play.

[1]S. A. Bingham et al., "Phytoestrogens: Where are we now?" *British Journal of Nutrition,* May 1998, 79(5) 393–406; S. T. Willard and L. S. Frawley. "Phytoestrogens have agonistic and combinatorial effects on estrogen-responsive gene expression in MCF-7 human breast cancer cells," *Endocrinology,* April 1998, 8(2), 117–121; T. B. Clarkson, "The potential of soybean phytoestrogens for postmenopausal hormone replacement therapy," *Proceedings of the Society of Experimental Biological Medicine,* March 1998, 217(3), 365–368.

Appendix A

Official Rules of Racquetball

1.0 The Game

1.1 Types of Games
1.2 Description
1.3 Objective
1.4 Points and Outs
1.5 Match, Game, Tiebreaker

2.0 Courts and Equipment

2.1 Court Specifications
2.2 Ball Specifications
2.3 Ball Selection
2.4 Racquet Specifications
2.5 Apparel

3.0 Play Regulations

3.1 Serve
3.2 Start
3.3 Manner
3.4 Readiness
3.5 Delays
3.6 Drive Service Zones
3.7 Defective Serves
3.8 Dead-Ball Serves
3.9 Fault Serves
3.10 Out Serves
3.11 Return of Serve
3.12 Changes of Serve
3.13 Rallies

D Procedures

FYI: Related Topics

Rulebook Index
ASTM Regulation Eyeguard List
Court Construction
Top of Document | USRA Homepage

1.0 The Game

Rule 1.1 TYPES OF GAMES
Racquetball is played by two or four players. When played by two, it is called singles and when played by four, doubles. A non-tournament variation of the game that is played by three players is called cut-throat.

Rule 1.2 DESCRIPTION
Racquetball is a competitive game in which a strung racquet is used to serve and return the ball.

Rule 1.3 OBJECTIVE
The objective is to win each rally by serving or returning the ball so the opponent is unable to keep the ball in play. A rally is over when a player (or team in doubles) is unable to hit the ball before it touches the floor twice, is unable to return the ball in such a manner that it touches the front wall before it touches the floor, or when a hinder is called.

Rule 1.4 POINTS AND OUTS
Points are scored only by the serving side when it serves an irretrievable serve (an ace) or wins a rally. Losing the serve is called a sideout in singles. In doubles, when the first server loses the serve it is called a handout and when the second server loses the serve it is a sideout.

Rule 1.5 MATCH, GAME, TIEBREAKER
A match is won by the first side winning two games. The first two games of a match are played to 15 points. If each side wins one game, a tiebreaker game is played to 11 points.

2.0 Courts and Equipment

Rule 2.1 COURT SPECIFICATIONS
The specifications for the standard four-wall racquetball court follow. (See also: construction specifications).

(a) Dimensions. The dimensions shall be 20 feet wide, 40 feet long and 20 feet high, with a back wall at least 12 feet high. All surfaces shall be in play, with the exception of any gallery opening, surfaces designated as out-of-play for a valid reason (such as being of a very different material or not in alignment with the backwall), and designated court hinders.

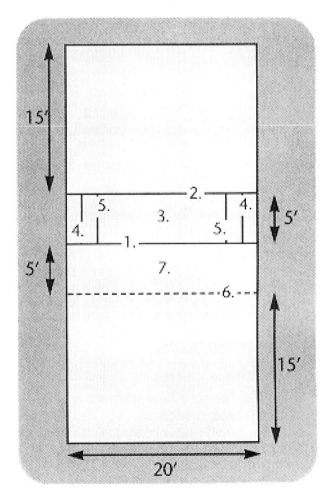

(b) Markings. Racquetball courts shall be marked with lines 1 1/2 inches wide as follows:

1. Short Line. The back edge of the short line is midway between, and is parallel with, the front and back walls.

2. Service Line. The front edge of the service line is parallel with, and five feet in front of, the back edge of the short line.

3. Service Zone. The service zone is the 5' × 20' area bounded by the bottom edges of the side walls and by the outer edges of the short line and the service line.

4. Service Boxes. The service boxes, used in doubles play, are located at each end of the service zone and are designated by lines parallel with the side walls [see 4.2(b)]. The edge of the line nearest to the center of the court shall be 18 inches from the nearest side wall.

5. Drive Serve Lines. The drive serve lines, which form the drive serve zone, are parallel with the side wall and are within the service zone. The edge of the line nearest to the center of the court shall be three feet from the nearest side wall.

6. Receiving Line. The receiving line is a broken line parallel to the short line. The back edge of the receiving line is five feet from the back edge of the short line. The receiving line begins with a line 21 inches long that extends from each side wall. These lines are connected by an alternate series of six-inch spaces and six-inch lines. This will result in a line composed of 17 six-inch spaces, 16 six-inch lines, and two 21-inch lines.

7. Safety Zone. The safety zone is the 5' × 20' area bounded by the bottom edges of the side walls and by the back edges of the short line and the receiving line. The zone is observed only during the serve. See Rules 3.10(i) and 3.11(a).

Rule 2.2 BALL SPECIFICATIONS

(a) The standard racquetball shall be 2 1/4 inches in diameter; weigh approximately 1.4 ounces; have a hardness of 55-60 inches durometer; and bounce 68-72 inches from a 100-inch drop at a temperature of 70-74 degrees Fahrenheit.

(b) Only a ball having the endorsement or approval of the USRA may be used in a USRA sanctioned tournament.

Rule 2.3 BALL SELECTION

(a) A ball shall be selected by the referee for use in each match. During the match the referee may, based on personal discretion or at the request of a player or team, replace the ball. Balls that are not round or which bounce erratically shall not be used.

(b) If possible, the referee and players should agree to an alternate ball, so that in the event of breakage, the second ball can be put into play immediately.

Rule 2.4 RACQUET SPECIFICATIONS

(a) The racquet, including bumper guard and all solid parts of the handle, may not exceed 22 inches in length.

(b) The racquet frame may be any material judged to be safe.

(c) The racquet frame must include a cord that must be securely attached to the player's wrist.

(d) The string of the racquet must be gut, monofilament, nylon, graphite, plastic, metal, or a combination thereof, and must not mark or deface the ball.

(e) Using an illegal racquet will result in forfeiture of the game in progress or, if discovered between games, forfeiture of the preceding game.

Rule 2.5 APPAREL

(a) All players must wear lensed eyewear that has been warranted by its manufacturer or distributor as 1.) designed for use in racquetball and 2.) meeting or exceeding either the full ASTM F803 standard or Canadian (CSA) impact standard. This rule applies to all persons, including those who wear corrective lenses. The eyewear must be unaltered and worn as designed at all times. A player who fails to wear proper eyewear will be assessed a technical foul and a timeout to obtain proper eyewear. A second infraction in the same match will result in immediate forfeiture of the match. [See Rule 3.17(a)9]

The USRA maintains a complete list of all eyewear so warranted by their manufacturers, and distributes the current list to the directors of every sanctioned event. In addition the list is published online at http://www.usra.org/pub&ref/eyeguard.htm, and may appear periodically in RACQUETBALL. A printed list is also made available upon request from the USRA's National Office [719/635-5396].

Eyewear not on the then-current list cannot be used in sanctioned events. An eyewear list with a date more than 60 days past the first day of the tournament will be deemed invalid for the purpose of determining compliance with this eyewear rule.

(b) Clothing and Shoes. The clothing may be of any color; however, a player may be required to change wet, extremely loose fitting, or otherwise distracting garments. Insignias and writing on the clothing must be considered to be in good taste by the tournament director. Shoes must have soles which do not mark or damage the floor.

(c) Equipment Requirements During Warm-up. Proper eyeguards [See Rule 2.5(a)] must be worn and wrist cords must be used during any on-court warm-up period. The referee should give a technical warning to any person who fails to comply and assess a technical foul if that player continues to not comply after receiving such a warning.

3.0 Play Regulations

Rule 3.1 SERVE

The server will have two opportunities to put the ball into play. The player or team winning the coin toss has the option to either serve or receive at the start of the first game. The second game will begin in reverse order of the first game. The player or team scoring the highest total of points in games 1 and 2 will have the option to serve or receive first at the start of the tiebreaker. In the event that both players or teams score an equal number of points in the first two games, another coin toss will take place and the winner of the toss will have the option to serve or receive.

Rule 3.2 START

The server may not start the service motion until the referee has called the score or "second serve." The serve is started from any place within the service zone. (Certain drive serves are an exception. See Rule 3.6.) Neither the ball nor any part of either foot may extend beyond either line of the service zone when initiating the service motion. Stepping on, but not beyond, the lines is permitted. However, when completing the service motion, the server may step beyond the service (front) line provided that some part of both feet remain on or inside the line until the served ball passes the short line. The server may not step beyond the short line until the ball passes the short line. See Rule 3.9(a) and 3.10(i) for penalties for violations.

Rule 3.3 MANNER

After taking a set position inside the service zone, a player may begin the service motion—any continuous movement which results in the ball being served. Once the service motion begins, the ball must be bounced on the floor in the zone and be struck by the racquet before it bounces a second time. After being struck, the ball must hit the front wall first and on the rebound hit the floor beyond the back edge of the short line, either with or without touching one of the side walls.

Rule 3.4 READINESS

The service motion shall not begin until the referee has called the score or the second serve and the server has visually checked the receiver. The referee shall call the score as both server and receiver prepare to return to their respective positions, shortly after the previous rally has ended.

Rule 3.5 DELAYS

Except as noted in Rule 3.5(b), the referee may call a technical foul for delays exceeding 10 seconds.

(a) The 10 second rule applies to the server and receiver simultaneously. Collectively, they are allowed up to 10 seconds after the score is called to serve or be ready to receive. It is the server's responsibility to look and be certain the receiver is ready. If a receiver is not ready, they must signal by raising the racquet above the head or completely turning the back to the server. (These are the only two acceptable signals.)

(b) Serving while the receiving player/team is signaling not ready is a fault serve.

(c) After the score is called, if the server looks at the receiver and the receiver is not signaling not ready, the server may then serve. If the receiver attempts to signal not ready after that point, the signal shall not be acknowledged and the serve becomes legal.

Rule 3.6 DRIVE SERVICE ZONES

The drive serve lines will be 3 feet from each side wall in the service zone. Viewed one at a time, the drive serve line divides the service area into a 3-foot and a 17-foot section that apply only to drive serves. The player may drive serve between the body and the side wall nearest to where the service motion began only if the player starts and remains outside of the 3-foot drive service zone. In the event that the service motion begins in one 3-foot drive service zone and continues into the other 3-foot drive serve zone, the player may not hit a drive serve at all.

(a) The drive serve zones are not observed for cross-court drive serves, the hard-Z, soft-Z, lob or half-lob serves.

(b) The racquet may not break the plane of the 17-foot zone while making contact with the ball.

(c) The drive serve line is not part of the 17-foot zone. Dropping the ball on the line or standing on the line while serving to the same side is an infraction.

Rule 3.7 DEFECTIVE SERVES
Defective serves are of three types resulting in penalties as follows:

(a) Dead-Ball Serve. A dead-ball serve results in no penalty and the server is given another serve (without canceling a prior fault serve).

(b) Fault Serve. Two fault serves result in an out (either a sideout or a handout).

(c) Out Serve. An out serve results in an out (either a sideout or a handout).

Rule 3.8 DEAD-BALL SERVES
Dead-ball serves do not cancel any previous fault serve. The following are dead-ball serves:

(a) Court Hinders. A serve that takes an irregular bounce because it hit a wet spot or an irregular surface on the court is a dead-ball serve. Also, any serve that hits any surface designated by local rules as an obstruction rather than being out-of-play.

(b) Broken Ball. If the ball is determined to have broken on the serve, a new ball shall be substituted and the serve shall be replayed, not canceling any prior fault serve.

Rule 3.9 FAULT SERVES
The following serves are faults and any two in succession result in an out:

(a) Foot Faults. A foot fault results when:

1. The server does not begin the service motion with both feet in the service zone.

2. The server steps completely over the service line (no part of the foot on or inside the service zone) before the served ball crosses the short line.

(b) Short Service. A short serve is any served ball that first hits the front wall and, on the rebound, hits the floor on or in front of the short line either with or without touching a side wall.

(c) Three Wall Serve. A three-wall serve is any served ball that first hits the front wall and, on the rebound, strikes both side walls before touching the floor.

(d) Ceiling Serve. A ceiling serve is any served ball that first hits the front wall and then touches the ceiling (with or without touching a side wall).

(e) Long Serve. A long serve is a served ball that first hits the front wall and rebounds to the back wall before touching the floor (with or without touching a side wall).

(f) Bouncing Ball Outside Service Zone. Bouncing the ball outside the service zone as a part of the service motion is a fault serve.

(g) Illegal Drive Serve. A drive serve in which the player fails to observe the 17-foot drive service zone outlined in Rule 3.6.

(h) Screen Serve. A served ball that first hits the front wall and on the rebound passes so closely to the server, or server's partner in doubles, that it prevents the receiver from having a clear view of the ball. (The receiver is obligated to take up good court position, near center court, to obtain that view.)

(i) Serving before the Receiver is Ready. A serve is made while the receiver is not ready as described in Rule 3.5(b).

Rule 3.10 OUT SERVES
Any of the following results in an out:

(a) Two Consecutive Fault Serves. See Rule 3.9.

(b) Missed Serve Attempt. Any attempt to strike the ball that results in a total miss or in the ball touching any part of the server's body. Also, allowing the ball to bounce more than once during the service motion.

(c) Touched Serve. Any served ball that on the rebound from the front wall touches the server or server's racquet before touching the floor, or any ball intentionally stopped or caught by the server or server's partner.

(d) Fake or Balk Serve. Any movement of the racquet toward the ball during the serve which is non-continuous and done for the purpose of deceiving the receiver. If a balk serve occurs, but the referee believes that no deceit was involved, the option of declaring "no serve" and having the serve replayed without penalty can be exercised.

(e) Illegal Hit. An illegal hit includes contacting the ball twice, carrying the ball, or hitting the ball with the handle of the racquet or part of the body or uniform.

(f) Non-Front Wall Serve. Any served ball that does not strike the front wall first.

(g) Crotch Serve. Any served ball that hits the crotch of the front wall and floor, front wall and side wall, or front wall and ceiling is an out serve (because it did not hit the front wall first). A serve into the crotch of the back wall and floor is a good serve and in play. A served ball that hits the crotch of the side wall and floor beyond the short line is in play.

(h) Out-of-Court Serve. An out-of-court serve is any served ball that first hits the front wall and, before striking the floor, either goes out of the court or hits a surface above the normal playing area of the court that has been declared as out-of-play for a valid reason [See Rule 2.1(a)].

(i) Safety Zone Violation. If the server, or doubles partner, enters into the safety zone before the served ball passes the short line, it shall result in the loss of serve.

Rule 3.11 RETURN OF SERVE
(a) Receiving Position
1. The receiver may not enter the safety zone until the ball bounces or crosses the receiving line.

2. On the fly return attempt, the receiver may not strike the ball until the ball breaks the plane of the receiving line. However, the receiver's follow-through may carry the receiver or the racquet past the receiving line.

3. Neither the receiver nor the racquet may break the plane of the short line, except if the ball is struck after rebounding off the back wall.

4. Any violation by the receiver results in a point for the server.

(b) Defective Serve. A player on the receiving side may not intentionally catch or touch a served ball (such as an apparently long or short serve) until the referee has made a call or the ball has touched the floor for a second time. Violation results in a point.

(c) Legal Return. After a legal serve, a player receiving the serve must strike the ball on the fly or after the first bounce, and before the ball touches the floor the second time; and return the ball to the front wall, either directly or after touching one or both side walls, the back wall or the ceiling, or any combination of those surfaces. A returned ball must touch the front wall before touching the floor.

(d) Failure to Return. The failure to return a serve results in a point for the server.

(e) Other Provisions. Except as noted in this rule (3.11), the return of serve is subject to all provisions of Rules 3.13 through 3.15.

Rule 3.12 CHANGES OF SERVE

(a) Outs. A server is entitled to continue serving until one of the following occurs:

1. Out Serve. See Rule 3.10.

2. Two Consecutive Fault Serves. See Rule 3.9.

3. Failure to Return Ball. Player or team fails to keep the ball in play as required by Rule 3.11(c).

4. Avoidable Hinder. Player or team commits an avoidable hinder which results in an out. See Rule 3.15.

(b) Sideout. Retiring the server in singles is called a sideout.

(c) Effect of Sideout. When the server (or serving team) receives a sideout, the server becomes the receiver and the receiver becomes the server.

Rule 3.13 RALLIES

All of the play which occurs after the successful return of serve is called the rally. Play shall be conducted according to the following rules:

(a) Legal Hits. Only the head of the racquet may be used at any time to return the ball. The racquet may be held in one or both hands. Switching hands to hit a ball, touching the ball with any part of the body or uniform, or removing the wrist safety cord during a rally results in a loss of the rally.

(b) One Touch. The player or team trying to return the ball may touch or strike the ball only once or else the rally is lost. The ball may not be carried. (A carried ball is one which rests on the racquet long enough that the effect is more of a sling or throw than a hit.)

(c) Failure to Return. Any of the following constitutes a failure to make a legal return during a rally:

1. The ball bounces on the floor more than once before being hit.

2. The ball does not reach the front wall on the fly.

3. The ball is hit such that it goes into the gallery or wall opening or else hits a surface above the normal playing area of the court that has been declared as out-of-play [See Rule 2.1(a)].

4. A ball which obviously does not have the velocity or direction to hit the front wall strikes another player.

5. A ball struck by one player on a team hits that player or that player's partner.

6. Committing an avoidable hinder. See Rule 3.15.

7. Switching hands during a rally.

8. Failure to use a racquet wrist safety cord.

9. Touching the ball with the body or uniform.

10. Carrying or slinging the ball with the racquet.

(d) Effect of Failure to Return. Violations of Rules 3.13 (a) through (c) result in a loss of rally. If the serving player or team loses the rally, it is an out. If the receiver loses the rally, it results in a point for the server.

(e) Return Attempts. The ball remains in play until it touches the floor a second time, regardless of how many walls it makes contact with—including the front wall. If a player swings at the ball and misses it, the player may continue to attempt to return the ball until it touches the floor for the second time.

(f) Broken Ball. If there is any suspicion that a ball has broken during a rally, play shall continue until the end of the rally. The referee or any player may request the ball be examined. If the referee decides the ball is broken the ball will be replaced and the rally replayed. The server will get two serves. The only proper way to check for a broken ball is to squeeze it by hand. (Checking the ball by striking it with a racquet will not be considered a valid check and shall work to the disadvantage of the player or team which struck the ball after the rally.)

(g) Play Stoppage

1. If a foreign object enters the court, or any other outside interference occurs, the referee shall stop the play immediately and declare a dead-ball hinder.

2. If a player loses any apparel, equipment, or other article, the referee shall stop play immediately and declare an avoidable hinder or dead-ball hinder as described in Rule 3.15(i).

(h) Replays. Whenever a rally is replayed for any reason, the server is awarded two serves. A previous fault serve is not considered.

Rule 3.14 DEAD-BALL HINDERS

A rally is replayed without penalty and the server resumes play at first serve whenever a dead-ball hinder occurs. Also, see Rule 3.15 which describes conditions under which a hinder might be declared avoidable and result in loss of the rally.

(a) Situations

1. Court Hinders. The referee should stop play immediately whenever the ball hits any part of the court that was designated in advance as a court hinder (such as a vent grate). The referee should also stop play

(i) when the ball takes an irregular bounce as a result of contacting a rough surface (such as court light or vent) or after striking a wet spot on the floor or wall and

(ii) when, in the referee's opinion, the irregular bounce affected the rally.

2. Ball Hits Opponent. When an opponent is hit by a return shot in flight, it is a dead-ball hinder. If the opponent is struck by a ball which obviously did not have the velocity or direction to reach the front wall, it is not a hinder, and the player who hit the ball will lose the rally. A player who has been hit by the ball can stop play and make the call though the call must be made immediately and acknowledged by the referee. Note this interference may, under certain conditions, be declared an avoidable hinder. See Rule 3.15.

3. Body Contact. If body contact occurs which the referee believes was sufficient to stop the rally, either for the purpose of preventing injury by further contact or because the contact prevented a player from being able to make a reasonable return, the referee shall call a hinder. Incidental body contact in which the offensive player clearly will have the advantage should not be called a hinder, unless the offensive player obviously stops play. Contact with the racquet on the follow-through normally is not considered a hinder.

4. Screen Ball. Any ball rebounding from the front wall so close to the body of the defensive player that it prevents the offensive player from having a clear view of the ball. (The referee should be careful not to make the screen call so quickly that it takes away a good offensive opportunity.) A ball that passes between the legs of a player who has just returned the ball is not automatically a screen. It depends on whether the other player is impaired as a result. Generally, the call should work to the advantage of the offensive player.

5. Backswing Hinder. Any body or racquet contact, on the backswing or on the way to or just prior to returning the ball, which impairs the hitter's ability to take a reasonable swing. This call can be made by the player attempting the return, though the call must be made immediately and is subject to the referee's approval. Note the interference may be considered an avoidable hinder. See Rule 3.15.

6. Safety Holdup. Any player about to execute a return who believes that striking the opponent with the ball or racquet is likely, may immediately stop play and request a dead-ball hinder. This call must be made immediately and is subject to acceptance and approval of the referee. (The referee will grant a dead-ball hinder if it is believed the holdup was reasonable and the player would have been able to return the shot. The referee may also call an avoidable hinder if warranted.)

7. Other Interference. Any other unintentional interference which prevents an opponent from having a fair chance to see or return the ball. Example: When a ball from another court enters the court during a rally or when a referee's call on an adjacent court obviously distracts a player.

(b) Effect of Hinders. The referee's call of hinder stops play and voids any situation which follows, such as the ball hitting the player. The only hinders that may be called by a player are described in rules (2), (5), and (6) above, and all of these are subject to the approval of the referee. A dead-ball hinder stops play and the rally is replayed. The server resumes play at first serve.

(c) Responsibility. While making an attempt to return the ball, a player is entitled to a fair chance to see and return the ball. It is the responsibility of the side that has just hit the ball to move so the receiving side may go straight to the ball and have an unobstructed view of and swing at the ball. However, the receiver is responsible for making a reasonable effort to move towards the ball and must have a reasonable chance to return the ball for any type of hinder to be called.

Rule 3.15 AVOIDABLE HINDERS
An avoidable hinder results in the loss of the rally. An avoidable hinder does not necessarily have to be an intentional act. Dead-ball hinders are described in Rule 3.14. Any of the following results in an avoidable hinder:

(a) Failure to Move. A player does not move sufficiently to allow an opponent a shot straight to the front wall as well as a cross-court shot which is a shot directly to the front wall at an angle that would cause the ball to rebound directly to the rear corner farthest from the player hitting the ball. Also when a player moves in such a direction that it prevents an opponent from taking either of these shots.

(b) Stroke Interference. This occurs when a player moves, or fails to move, so that the opponent returning the ball does not have a free, unimpeded swing. This includes unintentionally moving in a direction which prevents the opponent from making an open, offensive shot.

(c) Blocking. Moves into a position which blocks the opponent from getting to, or returning, the ball; or in doubles, a player moves in front of an opponent as the player's partner is returning the ball.

(d) Moving into the Ball. Moves in the way and is struck by the ball just played by the opponent.

(e) Pushing. Deliberately pushes or shoves opponent during a rally.

(f) Intentional Distractions. Deliberate shouting, stamping of feet, waving of racquet, or any other manner of disrupting one's opponent.

(g) View Obstruction. A player moves across an opponent's line of vision just before the opponent strikes the ball.

(h) Wetting the Ball. The players, particularly the server, should insure that the ball is dry prior to the serve. Any wet ball that is not corrected prior to the serve shall result in an avoidable hinder against the server.

(i) Apparel or Equipment Loss. If a player loses any apparel, equipment, or other article, play shall be immediately stopped and that player shall be called for an avoidable hinder, unless the player has just hit a shot that could not be retrieved. If the loss of equipment is caused by a player's opponent, then a dead-ball hinder should be called. If the opponent's action is judged to have been avoidable, then the opponent should be called for an avoidable hinder.

Rule 3.16 TIMEOUTS
(a) Rest Periods. Each player or team is entitled to three 30-second timeouts in games to 15 and two 30-second timeouts in games to 11. Timeouts may not be called by either side after service motion has begun. Calling for a timeout when none remain or after service motion has begun, or taking more than 30

seconds in a timeout, will result in the assessment of a technical foul for delay of game.

(b) Injury. If a player is injured during the course of a match as a result of contact, such as with the ball, racquet, wall or floor, an injury timeout will be awarded. While a player may call more than one timeout for the same injury or for additional injuries which occur during the match, a player is not allowed more than a total of 15 minutes of rest for injury during the entire match. If the injured player is not able to resume play after total rest of 15 minutes, the match shall be awarded to the opponent.

1. Should any external bleeding occur, the referee must halt play as soon as the rally is over, charge an injury timeout to the person who is bleeding, and not allow the match to continue until the bleeding has stopped.

2. Muscle cramps and pulls, fatigue, and other ailments that are not caused by direct contact on the court will not be considered an injury. Injury time is also not allowed for pre-existing conditions.

(c) Equipment Timeouts. Players are expected to keep all clothing and equipment in good, playable condition and are expected to use regular timeouts and time between games for adjustment and replacement of equipment. If a player or team is out of timeouts and the referee determines that an equipment change or adjustment is necessary for fair and safe continuation of the match, the referee may grant an equipment timeout not to exceed 2 minutes. The referee may allow additional time under unusual circumstances.

(d) Between Games. The rest period between the first two games of a match is 2 minutes. If a tiebreaker is necessary, the rest period between the second and third game is 5 minutes.

(e) Postponed Games. Any games postponed by referees shall be resumed with the same score as when postponed.

Rule 3.17 TECHNICAL FOULS AND WARNINGS

(a) Technical Fouls. The referee is empowered to deduct one point from a player's or team's score when, in the referee's sole judgment, the player is being overtly and deliberately abusive. If the player or team against whom the technical foul was assessed does not resume play immediately, the referee is empowered to forfeit the match in favor of the opponent. Some examples of actions which can result in technical fouls are:

1. Profanity.

2. Excessive arguing.

3. Threat of any nature to opponent or referee.

4. Excessive or hard striking of the ball between rallies.

5. Slamming of the racquet against walls or floor, slamming the door, or any action which might result in damage to the court or injury to other players.

6. Delay of game. Examples include

(i) taking too much time to dry the court,

(ii) excessive questioning of the referee about the rules,

(iii) exceeding the time allotted for timeouts or between games,

(iv) calling a timeout when none remain, or after the service motion begins, or

(v) taking more than ten seconds to serve or be ready to receive serve.

7. Intentional front line foot fault to negate a bad lob serve.

8. Anything the referee considers to be unsportsmanlike behavior.

9. Failure to wear lensed eyewear designed for racquet sports [See Rule 2.5(a)] is an automatic technical foul on the first infraction, plus a mandatory timeout (to acquire the proper eyewear) will be charged against the offending player. A second infraction by that player during the match will result in automatic forfeiture of the match.

(b) Technical Warnings. If a player's behavior is not so severe as to warrant a technical foul, a technical warning may be issued without the deduction of a point.

(c) Effect of Technical Foul or Warning. If a referee issues a technical foul, one point shall be removed from the offender's score. No point will be deducted if a referee issues a technical warning. In either case, a technical foul or warning should be accompanied by a brief explanation. Issuing a technical foul or warning has no effect on who will be serving when play resumes. If a technical foul occurs when the offender has no points or between games, the result will be that the offender's score becomes minus one (-1).

4.0-11.0 Rule Modifications

The following sections (4.0 through 11.0) detail the additional or modified rules that apply to variations of the singles game described in Sections 1 through 3.

4.0 Doubles

The USRA's rules for singles also apply in doubles with the following additions and modifications:

    4.1—Doubles Team

    4.2—Serve in Doubles

    4.3—Fault Serve in Doubles

    4.4—Out Serve in Doubles

    4.5—Return in Doubles

Rule 4.1 DOUBLES TEAM

(a) A doubles team shall consist of two players who meet either the age requirements or player classification requirements to participate in a particular division of play. A team with different skill levels must play in the division of the player with the higher level of ability. When playing in an adult age division, the team must play in the division of the younger player. When playing in a junior age division, the team must play in the division of the older player.

(b) A change in playing partners may be made so long as the first match of the posted team has not begun. For this purpose only, the match will be considered started once the teams have been called to the court. The team must notify the tournament director of the change prior to the beginning of the match.

Rule 4.2 SERVE IN DOUBLES

(a) Order of Serve. Each team shall inform the referee of the order of service which shall be followed throughout that game. The order of serve may be changed between games. At the beginning of each game, when the first server of the first team to serve is out, the team is out. Thereafter, both players on each team shall serve until the team receives a handout and a sideout.

(b) Partner's Position. On each serve, the server's partner shall stand erect with back to the side wall and with both feet on the floor within the service box from the moment the server begins the service motion until the served ball passes the short line. Violations are called foot faults. However, if the server's partner enters the safety zone before the ball passes the short line, the server loses service.

(c) Changes of Serve. In doubles, the side is retired when both partners have lost service, except that the team which serves first at the beginning of each game loses the serve when the first server is retired.

Rule 4.3 FAULT SERVE IN DOUBLES

(a) The server's partner is not in the service box with both feet on the floor and back to the side wall from the time the server begins the service motion until the ball passes the short line.

(b) A served ball that hits the doubles partner while in the doubles box results in a fault serve.

Rule 4.4 OUT SERVE IN DOUBLES

(a) Out-of-Order Serve. In doubles, when either partner serves out of order, the points scored by that server will be subtracted and an out serve will be called: if the second server serves out of order, the out serve will be applied to the first server and the second server will resume serving. If the player designated as the first server serves out of order, a sideout will be called. The referee should call "no serve" as soon as an out-of-order serve occurs. If no points are scored while the team is out of order, only the out penalty will have to be assessed. However, if points are scored before the out of order condition is noticed and the referee cannot recall the number, the referee may enlist the aid of the line judges (but not the crowd) to recall the number of points to be deducted.

(b) Ball Hits Partner. A served ball that hits the doubles partner while outside the doubles box results in loss of serve.

Rule 4.5 RETURN IN DOUBLES

(a) The rally is lost if one player hits that same player's partner with an attempted return.

(b) If one player swings at the ball and misses it, both partners may make further attempts to return the ball until it touches the floor the second time. Both partners on a side are entitled to return the ball.

5.0 One Serve

The USRA's standard rules governing racquetball play will be followed except for the following:

Rule 5.1 ONE SERVE
Only one serve is allowed. Therefore, any fault serve is an out serve, with a few exceptions.

Rule 5.2 SCREEN SERVE
If a serve is called a screen, the server will be allowed one more opportunity to hit a legal serve. Two consecutive screen serves results in an out.

Rule 5.3 SERVE HITS PARTNER
In doubles, if a serve hits the non-serving partner while standing in the box, the server will be allowed one more opportunity to hit a legal serve. Hitting the non-serving partner twice, results in an out.

Rule 5.4 CONSECUTIVE FAULTS
In doubles, either (i) a screen serve followed by hitting the non-serving partner or (ii) hitting the non-serving partner followed by a screen serve, results in an out.

6.0 Multi-Bounce

In general, the USRA's standard rules governing racquetball play will be followed except for the modifications which follow.

Rule 6.1 BASIC RETURN RULE
In general, the ball remains in play as long as it is bouncing. However, the player may swing only once at the ball and the ball is considered dead at the point it stops bouncing and begins to roll. Also, anytime the ball rebounds off the back wall, it must be struck before it crosses the short line on the way to the front wall, except as explained in Rule 6.2.

Rule 6.2 BLAST RULE
If the ball caroms from the front wall to the back wall on the fly, the player may hit the ball from any place on the court—including past the short line—so long as the ball is still bouncing.

Rule 6.3 FRONT WALL LINES
Two parallel lines (tape may be used) should be placed across the front wall such that the bottom edge of one line is 3 feet above the floor and the bottom edge of the other line is 1 foot above the floor. During the rally, any ball that hits the front wall
(i) below the 3-foot line and
(ii) either on or above the 1-foot line must be returned before it bounces a third time. However, if the ball hits below the 1-foot line, it must be returned before it bounces twice. If the ball hits on or above the 3-foot line, the ball must be returned as described in the basic return rule.

Rule 6.4 GAMES AND MATCHES
All games are played to 11 points and the first side to win two games, wins the match.

7.0 One-Wall & Three-Wall Play

In general, the USRA's standard rules governing racquetball play will be followed except for the modifications which follow.

Rule 7.1 ONE-WALL
There are two playing surfaces—the front wall and the floor. The wall is 20 feet wide and 16 feet high. The floor is 20 feet wide and 34 feet to the back edge of the long line. To permit movement by players, there should be a minimum of three feet (six feet is recommended) beyond the long line and six feet outside each side line.
    (a) Short Line. The back edge of the short line is 16 feet from the wall.
    (b) Service Markers. Lines at least six inches long which are parallel with, and midway between, the long and short lines. The extension of the service markers form the imaginary boundary of the service line.
    (c) Service Zone. The entire floor area inside and including the short line, side lines and service line.
    (d) Receiving Zone. The entire floor area in back of the short line, including the side lines and the long line.

Rule 7.2 THREE-WALL WITH SHORT SIDE WALL
The front wall is 20 feet wide and 20 feet high. The side walls are 20 feet long and 20 feet high, with the side walls tapering to 12 feet high. The floor length and court markings are the same as a four wall court.

Rule 7.3 THREE-WALL WITH LONG SIDE WALL
The court is 20 feet wide, 20 feet high and 40 feet long. The side walls may taper from 20 feet high at the front wall down to 12 feet high at the end of the court. All court markings are the same as a four wall court.

Rule 7.4 SERVICE IN THREE-WALL COURTS
A serve that goes beyond the side walls on the fly is an out. A serve that goes beyond the long line on a fly, but within the side walls, is a fault.

8.0 Wheelchair

Rule 8.1 CHANGES TO STANDARD RULES
In general, the USRA's standard rules governing racquetball play will be followed, except for the modifications which follow.
    (a) Where USRA rules refer to server, person, body, or other similar variations, for wheelchair play such reference shall include all parts of the wheelchair in addition to the person sitting on it.

(b) Where the rules refer to feet, standing or other similar descriptions, for wheelchair play it means only where the rear wheels actually touch the floor.

(c) Where the rules mention body contact, for wheelchair play it shall mean any part of the wheelchair in addition to the player.

(d) Where the rules refer to double bounce or after the first bounce, it shall mean three bounces. All variations of the same phrases shall be revised accordingly.

Rule 8.2 DIVISIONS

(a) Novice Division. The novice division is for the beginning player who is just learning to play.

(b) Intermediate Division. The Intermediate Division is for the player who has played tournaments before and has a skill level to be competitive in the division.

(c) Open Division. The Open Division is the highest level of play and is for the advanced player.

(d) Multi-Bounce Division. The Multi-Bounce Division is for the individuals (men or women) whose mobility is such that wheelchair racquetball would be impossible if not for the Multi-Bounce Division.

(e) Junior Division. The junior divisions are for players who are under the age of 19. The tournament director will determine if the divisions will be played as two bounce or multi-bounce. Age divisions are: 8–11, 12–15, and 16–18.

Rule 8.3 RULES

(a) Two Bounce Rule. Two bounces are used in wheelchair racquetball in all divisions except the Multi-Bounce Division. The ball may hit the floor twice before being returned.

(b) Out-of-Chair Rule. The player can neither intentionally jump out of the chair to hit a ball nor stand up in the chair to serve the ball. If the referee determines that the chair was left intentionally it will result in loss of the rally for the offender. If a player unintentionally leaves the chair, no penalty will be assessed. Repeat offenders will be warned by the referee.

(c) Equipment Standards. To protect playing surfaces, the tournament officials will not allow a person to participate with black tires or anything which will mark or damage the court.

(d) Start. The serve may be started from any place within the service zone. Although the front casters may extend beyond the lines of the service zone, at no time shall the rear wheels cross either the service or short line before the served ball crosses the short line. Penalties for violation are the same as those for the standard game.

(e) Maintenance Delay. A maintenance delay is a delay in the progress of a match due to a malfunction of a wheelchair, prosthesis, or assistive device. Such delay must be requested by the player, granted by the referee during the match, and shall not exceed 5 minutes. Only two such delays may be granted for each player for each match. After using both maintenance delays, the player has the following options:

(i) continue play with the defective equipment,

(ii) immediately substitute replacement equipment, or

(iii) postpone the game, with the approval of the referee and opponent.

Rule 8.4 MULTI-BOUNCE RULES

(a) The ball may bounce as many times as the receiver wants though the player may swing only once to return the ball to the front wall.

(b) The ball must be hit before it crosses the short line on its way back to the front wall.

(c) The receiver cannot cross the short line after the ball contacts the back wall.

9.0 Visually Impaired

In general, the USRA's standard rules governing racquetball play will be followed except for the modifications which follow.

Rule 9.1 ELIGIBILITY

A player's visual acuity must not be better than 20/200 with the best practical eye correction or else the player's field of vision must not be better than 20 degrees. The three classifications of blindness are B1 (totally blind to light perception), B2 (able to see hand movement up to 20/600 corrected), and B3 (from 20/600 to 20/200 corrected).

Rule 9.2 RETURN OF SERVE AND RALLIES

On the return of serve and on every return thereafter, the player may make multiple attempts to strike the ball until

(i) the ball has been touched,

(ii) the ball has stopped bouncing, or

(iii) the ball has passed the short line after touching the back wall. The only exception is described in Rule 9.3 below.

Rule 9.3 BLAST RULE

If the ball (other than on the serve) caroms from the front wall to the back wall on the fly, the player may retrieve the ball from any place on the court—including in front of the short line—so long as the ball has not been touched and is still bouncing.

Rule 9.4 HINDERS

A dead-ball hinder will result in the rally being replayed without penalty unless the hinder was intentional. If a hinder is clearly intentional, an avoidable hinder should be called and the rally awarded to the non-offending player or team.

10.0 Deaf

In general, the USRA's standard rules governing racquetball play will be followed except for the modifications which follow.

Rule 10.1 ELIGIBILITY
An athlete shall have a hearing loss of 55 db or more in the better ear to be eligible for any deaf tournament.

11.0 Professional

[IRT/Men & WIRT/Women]
In general, competition on both the International Racquetball Tour [IRT] and Women's International Racquetball Tour [WIRT] will follow the standard rules governing racquetball established by the USRA, except for the modifications which follow. Modifications for both professional tours are consistent, with one exception as noted in Rule 11.4.

Rule 11.1 GAME, MATCH
All games are played to 11 points, and are won by the player who scores to that level, with a 2-point lead. If necessary, the game will continue beyond 11 points, until such time as one player has a 2-point lead. Matches are played the best three out of a possible five games to 11.

Rule 11.2 APPEALS
The referee's call is final. There are no line judges, and no appeals may be made.

Rule 11.3 SERVE
Players are allowed only one serve to put the ball into play.

Rule 11.4 SCREEN SERVE
In IRT matches, screen serves are replayed. In WIRT matches, two consecutive screen serves will result in a sideout.

Rule 11.5 COURT HINDERS
No court hinders are allowed or called.

Rule 11.6 OUT-OF-COURT BALL
Any ball leaving the court results in a loss of rally.

Rule 11.7 BALL
All matches are played with the Penn Pro ball. The first, third, and fifth (if necessary) games of the match are started with a new ball.

Rule 11.8 TIMEOUTS
   (a) Per Game. Each player is entitled to one 1-minute timeout per game.
   (b) Between Points. The player has 15 seconds from the end of the previous rally to put the ball in play.
   (c) Between Games. The rest period between all games is 2 minutes, including a fifth game tiebreaker.
   (d) Equipment Timeouts. A player does not have to use regular timeouts to correct or adjust equipment, provided that the need for the change or adjustment is acknowledged by the referee as being necessary for fair and safe continuation of the match.

(e) Injury Timeout. Consists of two 7 1/2 minute timeouts within a match. Once an injury timeout is taken, the full 7 1/2 minutes must be used, or it is forfeited. Each player is entitled to one 1-minute timeout per game.

A—Tournaments
A.1 Draws

(a) If possible, all draws shall be made at least two (2) days before the tournament commences. The seeding method of drawing shall be approved by the USRA.

(b) At USRA National events, the draw and seeding committee shall be chaired by the USRA's Executive Director, National Tournament Director, and the host tournament director. No other persons shall participate in the draw or seeding unless at the invitation of the draw and seeding committee.

(c) In local and regional tournaments the draw shall be the responsibility of the tournament director.

A.2 Consolation Matches

(a) Each entrant shall be entitled to participate in a minimum of two matches. Therefore, losers of their first match shall have the opportunity to compete in a consolation bracket of their own division. In draws of less than seven players, a round robin may be offered. See A.6 about how to determine the winner of a round robin event.

(b) Consolation matches may be waived at the discretion of the tournament director, but this waiver must be in writing on the tournament application.

(c) Preliminary consolation matches will be two of three games to 11 points. Semifinal and final matches will follow the regular scoring format.

A.3 Scheduling

(a) Preliminary Matches. If one or more contestants are entered in both singles and doubles, they may be required to play both singles and doubles on the same day with little rest between matches. This is a risk assumed on entering two singles events or a singles and doubles event. If possible, the schedule should provide at least 1 hour of rest between matches.

(b) Final Matches. Where one or more players has reached the finals in both singles and doubles, it is recommended that the doubles match be played on the day preceding the singles. This would assure more rest between the final matches. If both final matches must be played on the same day or night, the following procedure is recommended:

(1) The singles match be played first, and;

(2) A rest period of not less than 1 hour be allowed between the finals in singles and doubles.

A.4 Notice of Matches

After the first round of matches, it is the responsibility of each player to check the posted schedules to determine the time and place of each subsequent match. If any change is made in the schedule after posting, it shall be the duty of the tournament director to notify the players of the change.

A.5 Third Place

Players are not required to play off for third place. However, for point standings, if one semifinalist wants to play off for third and the other semifinalist does not, the one willing to play shall be awarded third place. If neither semifinalist wishes to play off for 3rd then the points shall be totaled, divided by 2, and awarded evenly to both players.

A.6 Round Robin Scoring

The final positions of players or teams in round robin competition is determined by the following sequence:

a. Winner of the most matches;

b. In a two way tie, winner of the head-to-head match;

c. In a tie of three or more, the player who lost the fewest games is awarded the highest position.

1. If a two way tie remains, the winner of the head-to-head match is awarded the higher position.

2. If a multiple tie remains, the total "points scored against" each player in all matches will be tabulated and the player who had the least "points scored against" them is awarded the highest position.

Note: Forfeits will count as a match won in two games. In cases where "points scored against" is the tiebreaker, the points scored by the forfeiting team will be discounted from consideration of "points scored against" all teams.

A.7 Court Assignments

In all USRA sanctioned tournaments, the tournament director and/or USRA official in attendance may decide on a change of court after the completion of any tournament game, if such a change will accommodate better spectator conditions.

A.8 Tournament Conduct

In all USRA sanctioned tournaments, the referee is empowered to forfeit a match, if the conduct of a player or team is considered detrimental to the tournament and the game. See B.5(d) and B.5(e).

B—Officiating

B.1 Tournament Management

All USRA sanctioned tournaments shall be managed by a tournament director, who shall designate the officials.

B.2 Tournament Rules Committee

The tournament director should appoint a tournament rules committee to resolve any disputes that the referee, tournament desk, or tournament director cannot resolve. The committee, composed of an odd number of persons, may include state or national officials, or other qualified individuals in attendance who are prepared to meet on short notice. The tournament director should not be a member of this committee.

B.3 Referee Appointment and Removal

The principal official for every match shall be the referee who has been designated by the tournament director, or a designated representative, and who has been agreed upon by all participants in the match. The referee's authority regarding a match begins once the players are called to the court. The referee may be removed from a match upon the agreement of all participants (teams in doubles) or at the discretion of the tournament director or the designated representative. In the event that a referee's removal is requested by one player or team and not agreed to by the other, the tournament director or the designated representative may accept or reject the request. It is suggested that the match be observed before determining what, if any, action is to be taken. In addition, two line judges and a scorekeeper may also be designated to assist the referee in officiating the match.

B.4 Rules Briefing

Before all tournaments, all officials and players shall be briefed on rules as well as local court hinders, regulations, and modifications the tournament director wishes to impose. The briefing should be reduced to writing. The current USRA rules will apply and be made available. Any modifications the tournament director wishes to impose must be stated on the entry form and be available to all players at registration.

B.5 Referees

(a) Pre-Match Duties. Before each match begins, it shall be the duty of the referee to:

1. Check on adequacy of preparation of court with respect to cleanliness, lighting and temperature.

2. Check on availability and suitability of materials to include balls, towels, scorecards, pencils and timepiece necessary for the match.

3. Check the readiness and qualifications of the line judges and scorekeeper. Review appeal procedures and instruct them of their duties, rules and local regulations.

4. Go onto the court to make introductions; brief the players on court hinders (both designated and undesignated); identify any out-of-play areas [see Rule 2.1(a)]; discuss local regulations and rule modifications for this tournament; and explain often misinterpreted rules.

5. Inspect players' equipment; identify the line judges; verify selection of a primary and alternate ball.

6. Toss coin and offer the winner the choice of serving or receiving.

(b) Decisions. During the match, the referee shall make all decisions with regard to the rules. Where line judges are used, the referee shall announce all final judgments. If both players in singles and three out of four in a doubles match disagree with a call made by the referee, the referee is overruled, with the exception of technical fouls and forfeitures.

(c) Protests. Any decision of the referee will, on protest, be accorded due process as set forth in the constitution of the USRA. For the purposes of rendering a prompt decision regarding protests filed during the course of an ongoing tournament, the stages of due process will be: first to the tournament desk, then to the tournament director, and finally to the tournament rules committee. In those instances when time permits, the protest may be elevated to the state association or, when appropriate, to the national level as called for in the USRA constitution.

(d) Forfeitures. A match may be forfeited by the referee when:

1. Any player refuses to abide by the referee's decision or engages in unsportsmanlike conduct.

2. Any player or team who fails to report to play 10 minutes after the match has been scheduled to play. (The tournament director may permit a longer delay if circumstances warrant such a decision.) A game will be forfeited by the referee for using an illegal racquet as specified in Rule 2.4(e).

(e) Defaults. A player or team may be forfeited by the tournament director or official for failure to comply with the tournament or host facility's rules while on the premises between matches, or for abuse of hospitality, locker room, or other rules and procedures.

(f) Spectators. The referee shall have jurisdiction over the spectators, as well as the players, while the match is in progress.

(g) Other Rulings. The referee may rule on all matters not covered in the USRA Official Rules. However, the referee's ruling is subject to protest as described in B.5(c).

B.6 Line Judges

(a) When Utilized. Two line judges should be used for semifinal and final matches, when requested by a player or team, or when the referee or tournament director so desires. However, the use of line judges is subject to availability and the discretion of the tournament director.

(b) Replacing Line Judges. If any player objects to a person serving as a line judge before the match begins, all reasonable effort shall be made to find a replacement acceptable to the officials and players. If a player objects after the match begins, any replacement shall be at the discretion of the referee and/or tournament director.

(c) Position of Line Judges. The players and referee shall designate the court location of the line judges. Any dispute shall be settled by the tournament director.

(d) Duties and Responsibilities. Line judges are designated to help decide appeals. In the event of an appeal, and after a very brief explanation of the appeal by the referee, the line judges must indicate their opinion of the referee's call.

(e) Signals. Line judges should extend their arm and signal as follows:

(i) thumb up to show agreement with the referee's call,

(ii) thumb down to show disagreement, and

(iii) hand open with palm facing down to indicate "no opinion" or that the play in question wasn't seen.

(f) Manner of Response. Line judges should be careful not to signal until the referee announces the appeal and asks for a ruling. In responding to the referee's request, line judges should not look at each other, but indicate their opinions simultaneously in clear view of the players and referee. If at any time a line judge is unsure of which call is being appealed or what the referee's call was, the line judge should ask the referee to repeat the call and the appeal.

(g) Result of Response. The referee's call stands if at least one line judge agrees with the referee or if neither line judge has an opinion. If both line judges disagree with the referee, the referee must reverse the call. If one line judge disagrees with the referee and the other signals no opinion, the rally is replayed. Any replays, with the exception of appeals on the second serve itself, will result in two serves.

B.7 Appeals

(a) Appealable Calls and Non-Calls. In any match using line judges, a player may appeal any call or non-call by the referee, except for a technical foul or forfeiture.

(b) How to Appeal. A verbal appeal by a player must be made directly to the referee immediately after the rally has ended. A player who believes there is an infraction to appeal, should bring it to the attention of the referee and line judges by raising the nonracquet hand at the time the perceived infraction occurs. The player is obligated to continue to play until the rally has ended or the referee stops play. The referee will recognize a player's appeal only if it is made before that player leaves the court for any reason including timeouts and game-ending rallies or, if that player doesn't leave the court, before the next serve begins.

(c) Loss of Appeal. A player or team forfeits its right of appeal for that rally if the appeal is made directly to the line judges or, if the appeal is made after an excessive demonstration or complaint.

(d) Limit on Appeals. A player or team can make three appeals per game. However, if either line judge disagrees (thumb down) with the referee's call, that appeal will not count against the three-appeal limit. In addition, a potential game-ending rally may be appealed without charge against the limit—even if the three-appeal limit has been reached.

B.8 Outcome of Appeals

Everything except technical fouls and forfeitures can be appealed. The following outcomes cover several of the most common types of appeal, but not all possible appeals could be addressed. Therefore, referee's discretion and common sense should govern the outcomes of those appeals that are not covered herein:

(a) Skip Ball. If the referee makes a call of "skip ball," and the call is reversed, the referee then must decide if the shot in question could have been returned had play continued. If, in the opinion of the referee, the shot could have been returned, the rally shall be replayed. However, if the shot was not retrievable, the side which hit the shot in question is declared the winner of the rally. If the referee makes no call on a shot (thereby indicating that the shot did not skip), an appeal may be made that the shot skipped. If the "no call" is reversed, the side which hit the shot in question loses the rally.

(b) Fault Serve. If the referee makes a call of fault serve and the call is reversed, the serve is replayed, unless if the referee considered the serve to be not retrievable, in which case a point is awarded to the server. If an appeal is made because the referee makes no call on a serve—thereby indicating that the serve was good—and the "no call" is reversed, it will result in second serve if the infraction occurred on the first serve or loss of serve if the infraction occurred on the second serve.

(c) Out Serve. If the referee calls an "out serve", and the call is reversed, the serve will be replayed, unless the serve was obviously a fault too, in which case the call becomes fault serve. However, if the call is reversed and the serve was considered an ace, a point will be awarded. Also, if the referee makes no call on a serve—thereby indicating that the serve was good—but the "no call" is reversed, it results in an immediate loss of serve.

(d) Double Bounce Pickup. If the referee makes a call of two bounces, and the call is reversed, the rally is replayed, except if the player against whom the call was made hit a shot that could not have been retrieved, then that player wins the rally. (Before awarding a rally in this situation, the referee must be certain that the shot would not have been retrieved even if play had not been halted.) If an appeal is made because the referee makes no call thereby indicating that the get was not two bounces, and the "no call" is reversed, the player who made the two bounce pickup is declared the loser of the rally.

(e) Receiving Line Violation (Encroachment). If the referee makes a call of encroachment, but the call is overturned, the serve shall be replayed unless the return was deemed irretrievable in which case a sideout (or possibly a handout in doubles) should be called. When an appeal is made because the referee made no call, and the appeal is successful, the server is awarded a point.

(f) Court Hinder. If the referee makes a call of court hinder during a rally or return of serve, the rally is replayed. If the referee makes no call and a player feels that a court hinder occurred, that player may appeal. If the appeal is successful, the rally will be replayed. A court hinder on a second serve results in only that serve being replayed.

B.9 Rule Interpretations

If a player feels the referee has interpreted the rules incorrectly, the player may require the referee or tournament director to cite the applicable rule in the rulebook. Having discovered a misapplication or misinterpretation, the official must correct the error by replaying the rally, awarding the point, calling sideout, or taking other corrective measures.

C—Eligibility and National Events

C.1 Professional

A professional is defined as any player who has accepted prize money regardless of the amount in any professional sanctioned (including IRT/WIRT) tournament or in any other tournament so deemed by the USRA Board of Directors. (NOTE: Any player concerned about the adverse effect of losing amateur status should contact the USRA National Office at the earliest opportunity to ensure a clear understanding of this rule and that no action is taken that could jeopardize that status.)

(a) An amateur player may participate in a professional sanctioned tournament but will not be considered a professional

(i) if no prize money is accepted or

(ii) if the prize money received remains intact and placed in trust under USRA guidelines.

(b) The acceptance of merchandise or travel expenses shall not be considered prize money, and thus does not jeopardize a player's amateur status.

C.2 Return to Amateur Status

Any player who has been classified as a professional can re-establish amateur status by requesting, in writing, this desire to be reclassified as an amateur. This application shall be tendered to the Executive Director of the USRA or a designated representative, and shall become effective immediately as long as the player making application for reinstatement of amateur status has received no money in any tournament, as defined in C.1, for the past 12 months.

C.3 USRA Eligibility

(a) Any current USRA member who has not been classified as a professional (See C.1) may compete in any USRA sanctioned tournament.

(b) Any current USRA member who has been classified as a professional may compete in any event at a USRA sanctioned tournament that offers prize money or merchandise.

(c) Amateur Athletic Waiver and Release of Liability. In consideration of being allowed to participate in any United States Racquetball Association athletics/sports programs, and related events and activities, all member signators:

1. Agree that prior to participating, they will inspect the facilities and equipment to be used, and if they believe anything is unsafe, they will immediately advise their coach, supervisor, or USRA personnel of such condition(s) and refuse to participate.

2. Acknowledge and fully understand that each participant will be engaging in activities that involve risk of serious injury, including permanent disability and death, and severe social and economic losses which might result not only from their own actions, inactions of negligence but the actions, inactions or negligence of others, the rules of play, or the condition of the premises or of any equipment used. Further, that there may be other risks not known to us or not reasonably foreseeable at this time.

3. Assume all the foregoing risks and accept personal responsibility for the damages following such injury, permanent disability or death.

4. Release, waive, discharge and covenant not to sue the United States Racquetball Association, its affiliated clubs, regional sports organizations, their respective administrators, directors, agents, coaches, and other employees of the organization, other participants, sponsoring agencies, sponsors, advertisers, and, if applicable, owners and lessees of premises used to conduct the event, all of which are hereinafter referred to as "releasees" from any and all liability to the signator on the opposite side of this form, his or her heirs and next of kin for any and all claims, demands, losses or damages on account of injury including death or damage to property, caused or alleged to be caused in whole or in part by the negligence of the release of otherwise.

C.4 Recognized Divisions

Title opportunities at national championships will be selected from the division lists which follow. Combined "Age + Skill" divisions may also be offered to provide additional competitive opportunities for non-open entrants. For ranking consistency, state organizations are encouraged to select from these recognized divisions when establishing competition in all sanctioned events.

(a) Open Division. Any player with amateur status.

(b) Open Adult Age Divisions. Eligibility is determined by the player's age on the first day of the tournament. Divisions are:

24 & under Varsity
25 + Junior Veterans
30+ Veterans
35+ Seniors
40+ Veteran Seniors
45+ Masters
50+ Veteran Masters
55+ Golden Masters
60+ Veteran Golden Masters
65+ Senior Golden Masters
70+ Advanced Golden Masters
75+ Super Golden Masters
80+ Grand Masters
85+ Super Grand Masters

(c) Junior Age Divisions. Player eligibility is determined by the player's age on January 1st of the current calendar year. Divisions are:

18 & Under
16 & Under
14 & Under
12 & Under
10 & Under
8 & Under (regular rules)
8 & Under (multi-bounce rules)
6 & Under (regular rules)
6 & Under (multi-bounce rules)

(d) Skill Divisions. Player eligibility is determined by AmPRO skill level certification, or verification by a state association official, at the entered level.

Elite [Open level drop-down only]
A
B
C
D
Novice

(e) Age + Skill Divisions. Player eligibility is determined by the player's age on the first day of the tournament, plus AmPRO skill level certification, or verification by a state association official, at the entered level. Such combinations may be offered as additional competition to players who do not fall into the "open" or designated skill levels of play. For example: 24− A/B, 30+ B, 35+ C/D, 40+ A, 65 + A/B, etc.

C.5 Division Competition by Gender

Men and women may compete only in events and divisions for their respective gender during regional and national tournaments. If there is not sufficient number of players to warrant play in a specific division, the tournament director may place the entrants in a comparably competitive division. Note: For the purpose of encouraging the development of women's racquetball, the governing bodies of numerous states permit women to play in men's divisions when a comparable skill level is not available in the women's divisions.

C.6 USRA Regional Championships

(a) Adult Regional Tournaments

1. Regional tournaments will be conducted at various metropolitan sites designated annually by the USRA and players may compete at any site they choose.

2. A person may compete in any number of adult regional tournaments, but may not enter a championship division (as listed in C.4) after having won that division at a previous adult regional tournament that same year.

3. A person cannot participate in more than two championship events at a regional tournament.

4. Any awards or remuneration to a USRA National Championship will be posted on the entry blank.

5. One-serve rules (see Rule 5.0) will be used in all open divisions at USRA National and Regional Championships. Their use is optional at other tournaments.

(b) Junior Regional Tournaments. Separate regional qualifying events for juniors have been discontinued. In order to qualify for annual Junior National events, players must compete in a sanctioned Level Three State Championship.

C.7 U.S. National Singles and Doubles Championships

The U.S. National Singles and Doubles Tournaments are separate tournaments and are played on different dates. One serve rules (see Rule 5.0) will apply in all Open divisions. National Singles are traditionally held in May; National Doubles in October.

(a) Competition in an Adult Regional singles tournament (or recognized qualifying event) is required to qualify for the National Singles Championship.

1. Recognized qualifying events are:
WSMA Championships (January)
NMRA Singles Championships (February)
World Intercollegiate Championships (April)

(b) The National Tournament Director may handle the rating of each region and determine how many players shall qualify from each regional tournament.

C.8 U.S. National Junior Olympic Championships

It will be conducted on a different date than all other National Championships. Traditionally held in June.

C.9 U.S. National High School Championships

It will be conducted on a different date than all other National Championships. Traditionally held in March.

C.10 World Intercollegiate Championships

It will be conducted on a different date than all other National Championships. Traditionally held in March/April.

C.11 U.S. Open Racquetball Championships

It will be conducted on a different date than all other National Championships, and include both pro and amateur competitive divisions. Traditionally held in November/December.

D—Procedures

D.1 Rule Change Procedures

To ensure the orderly growth of racquetball, the USRA has established specific procedures that are followed before a major change is made to the rules of the game. NOTE: Changes to rules and regulations in Sections 1 through 10 must adhere to published rule change procedures. Remaining sections may be altered by vote of the USRA Board of Directors.

1. Rule change proposals must be submitted in writing to the USRA National Office by June 1st. NOTE: The Board of Directors has imposed a moratorium on rule changes that establishes the next deadline for submission of rule change proposals as June 1, 2001, which would set the earliest possible effective date as September 1, 2002. [See following timeline for procedural details.]

2. The USRA Board of Directors will review all proposals at its October board meeting and determine which will be considered.

3. Selected proposals will appear in RACQUETBALL Magazine—the official USRA publication—as soon as possible after the October meeting for comment by the general membership.

4. After reviewing membership input and the recommendations of the National Rules Committee and National Rules Commissioner, the proposals are discussed and voted upon at the annual Board of Directors meeting in May.

5. Changes approved in May become effective on September 1st. Exception: changes in racquet specifications become effective two years later on September 1st.

6. Proposed rules that are considered for adoption in one year, but are not approved by the Board of Directors in May of that year, will not be considered for adoption the following year.

The following "policies & procedures" segments are subject to stated rule change procedures outlined in D.1:

A.6 Round Robin Scoring
A.8 Tournament Conduct
B.5 (d-g) Forfeitures, Defaults . . .
B.6 Line Judges
B.7 Appeals
B.8 Outcome of Appeals

D.2 USRA National Rules Committee

Rich Clay, National Rules Commissioner
3401 North Kedzie
Chicago, IL 60618
773/539-1114 (Office)
847/918-7407 (Home)

Michael Arnolt
Suite 307 3833 North Meridian Street
Indianapolis, IN 46208
317/926-2766 (Office)
317/259-1359 (Home)

Dan J. Davis
5304 Hollister Street
Houston, TX 77040
817/666-9139 (Office)

Otto Dietrich
4244 Russet Court
Lilburn, GA 30047
770/972-2303 (Home)

Jim Easterling
321 Village Lansing, MI 48911
517/887-0459 (Home)
517/373-2399 (Office)

Lorraine Galloway
175-20 Wexford Terrace #7-5
Jamaica Estates, NY 11432
718/739-4629 (Home)

Jim Gillhouse
2120 East Willamette Avenue
Colorado Springs, CO 80909
719/471-0799 (Home)
719/526-9636 (Office)

Mary Lyons
940 Penman Road
Neptune Beach, FL 32266
904/241-6789 (Home)

Eric Muller
445 Fifth Avenue, Apt. 32-C
New York, NY 10016
212/683-1610 (Home)

Annie Muniz
812 Woodstock Bellaire, TX 77401
713/659-3554 (Office)
713/432-0881 (Home)

Appendix B

Racquetball Associations

United States Racquetball Association
1685 West Uintah
Colorado Springs, CO 80904
719-635-5396

IRT/WIRT (International Racquetball Tour/Women's International Racquetball
    Tour)
13735 Regency Ct.
Lake Oswego, OR 97035
Hank Marcus

Appendix C

Manufacturers of Racquetball Equipment

For general information:

Racquetball Manufacturers Association
200 Castlewood Drive
North Palm Beach, FL 33408
(407) 842-4100

For specific manufacturers:

Ashaway
24 Laurel Street
Ashaway, RI 02804
(800) 556-7260
ashawaysales@edgenet.net

E-Force
7920 Arjons Dr. Unit A
San Diego, CA 92126
(800) 433-6723

Ektelon
One Sportsystem Plaza
Bordentown, NJ 08505
(800) 283-6647

Head-Penn Racquet Sports
306 So. 45th Ave.
Phoenix, AZ 85043
(602) 269-1492

Leader Sports Products
60 Lakeshore Road
Essex, NY 12936
(800) 363-5546
swinters@headUSA.com

Pro Kennex
9606 Kearny Villa Road
San Diego, CA 92126-4589
(800) 854-1908
infopk@prokennex.com

Python Racquetball
205 Axton Ct.
Roswell, GA 30076
(770) 751-9463
python2@mindspring.com

Wilson Racquet Sports
8700 W. Bryn Mawr Ave.
Chicago, IL 60631
(773) 714-6720
terrigraham@racquet.wilsonsports.com

Glossary

Ace A legal serve that is not returned by the receiver; garners a point for the server.

Alley An imaginary lane along both side walls that is the target area for down-the-line shots.

Anticipating Predicting your opponent's next shot.

Apex The highest point of a ball's bounce.

Appeal When a player asks the line judges to reverse the referee's decision on an appealable call.

Around-the-wall shot A defensive shot that hits a side wall, the front wall, and then the other side wall.

Avoidable hinder Occurs when a player interferes with the shooter's shot in a manner that was preventable; results in a point or a side out for the opponent. Does not necessarily have to be intentional.

Back court The area of the court from the back wall to the receiving line.

Backhand The stroke used when the ball is hit on the side of the body opposite the racquet hand.

Back into back wall shot A defensive shot hit into the back wall hard enough for it to rebound to the front wall. This is a shot made as a last resort.

Backspin Hitting the ball so that it spins backward, with the under part of the ball moving forward, slowing the ball's flight.

Backswing Bringing the racquet back in preparation for a forward stroke.

Backswing hinder Occurs when a player interferes with or blocks the path of the backswing. Contact is not necessary.

Back wall The rear wall.

Backwall shot Hitting a ball that has rebounded from the back wall on its way toward the front wall.

BB backwall shot A shot hit high on the front wall that goes directly to the back wall and then hits the floor.

Block Using one's body to impede an opponent's progress toward the ball; a hinder.

Body contact Bumping, colliding with, or touching an opponent. Usually grounds for a hinder.

Boron A material used in high-tech racquets, usually as a composite with graphite.

Bottom board The lowest point on the front wall; the target for kill shots.

Bumper guard Plastic protective covering on the outside rim of a racquet head; prevents damage to the racquet.

Butt The end of the racquet handle.

Bye When a player does not have to play a match in the first round of a tournament in order to advance to the second round.

Ceiling serve A fault serve that hits the ceiling after it hits the front wall.

Ceiling shot A defensive shot that hits the ceiling before the front wall. It should land deep in the back court.

Center court The area of the court immediately behind the short service line and in the middle of the court. Controlling this area gives the greatest advantage for control of the game.

Change of pace A shot in which the speed is changed from that which is normal (usually slower than normal).

Composite A blending of materials used in racquet construction.

Consolation round A tournament for those who have been defeated in the first round of a tournament. This enables losers to play others who have lost.

Controlling center court Occurs when a player plays in the center court area, which usually forces the other player to play in the back court.

Court hinder When the path of the ball has been affected by objects or areas on the court; calls for replaying the point.

Cross-court pass shot A shot from one side of the court that passes the opponent on the opposite side; should be hit at knee level.

Crotch ball A shot that hits directly at the juncture point of any two surfaces (walls, floor, ceiling).

Crotch serve Considered an out serve.

Crowding Not giving one's opponent enough room to play a shot; a hinder.

Cutthroat A game with three players, in which the server plays against the other two players.

Dead ball A ball no longer in play.

Dead ball serve A serve that incurs no penalty and is played over. It can be caused by a court hinder, a broken ball, or the ball hitting the server's partner while in the service box.

Default The termination of a game when one player cannot or will not continue.

Defective serve Any illegal serve, dead ball serve, fault serve, or out serve.

Defensive shot Any shot in which the objective is other than terminating the rally. Examples are ceiling, around-the-wall, and "Z" shots.

Die A ball that loses momentum and drops suddenly.

Dig Saving a shot by playing it just before it takes a second bounce.

Donut A game in which the losing player does not score a point (a shutout).

Double bounce When the ball hits the floor twice before being returned; results in a point or side out.

Doubles A game involving two teams of two players each.

Down-the-wall pass A shot that passes the opponent on the same side of the court on which the ball was hit, parallel to the wall.

Draw Selection of the positions in which players will be placed in a tournament.

Drive serve A hard-hit, low serve.

Drive service zone Area in the service zone between a side wall and the three-foot line.

Drop shot A soft, easy shot that rebounds only a short distance off the front wall.

Error Missing an easy shot that should have been hit.

Fault serve An illegal serve, such as: short serve, long serve, ceiling serve, three-wall serve, out-of-court serve, foot fault, screen serve, and missed serve. Two consecutive faults result in loss of service.

Fly shot A shot returned directly from the front wall before it hits the floor.

Follow-through The completion of the swinging action after the ball has been hit.

Foot fault Illegal serve in which a server's foot touches the area outside of the service area during a serve, or, in doubles, when the server's partner is not in the service box during the serve.

Footwork Proper positioning of the feet to get to a shot or to make a specific shot.

Forehand A shot hit on the racquet-hand side of the body.

Forfeit A loss for a player who does not appear for a tournament game.

Front and back A system of doubles play in which one partner plays up and the other back; the I formation.

Front court The part of the court from the front wall to the service line.

Front wall kill A hard, low shot that hits only the front wall before bouncing.

Game When one team or player reaches 15 points (or the agreed-on number of points).

Game Point When the server is going for the point that will win the game.

Garbage serve A half-lob serve that reaches the opponent at shoulder height.

Graphite A material used in manufacturing racquets, often in combination with other materials (a composite).

Grip Position of the hand on the racquet.

Half and half An alignment of the partners in doubles in which each covers half of the court, from front wall to back wall. (side by side)

Half volley Hitting the ball just after it has bounced.

Hand One player's service turn.

Hand out When one player loses service in a doubles game.

Head of the racquet The hitting area of the racquet, which contains the strings.

Hinder Interference with a player's opportunity to get a clean shot at the ball. If a hinder is called, the point is replayed.

Hit opponent When the ball hits an opponent; results in a hinder if the ball is going toward the front wall, and ends a rally if the ball is returning from the front wall.

I formation Strategy of doubles play in which one player is responsible for the front court and the other takes the back court.

Illegal hit Occurs when the ball contacts any part of a player or a player's uniform; treated as an out serve or the end of the rally.

Jam serve A serve that is directed at the opponent's body, forcing the opponent to move.

Kill shot An offensive shot hit hard and low, which should bounce twice before the opponent has a chance to return it.

Line judge Helps decide appeal calls. Two line judges can overrule the referee on appealable calls.

Live ball A ball in play.

Lob serve A high serve that rebounds in a high arc, landing just short of the back wall.

Lob shot A soft shot hit high on the front wall that will rebound high and to the back court.

Long serve A fault serve that hits the back wall before the floor.

Macro An oversized racquet with a larger-than-normal head.

Masters division A competitive division for players who are at least 45 years old.

Match When one player or team wins two out of three games.

Match point When the serving player or team is going for the point that will win the match.

Mid-court The area between the service line and the receiving line.

Mixed doubles Doubles play in which each team is composed of a male and a female player.

Non-front serve An out serve that hits the floor, ceiling, or a side wall before making contact with the front wall; results in loss of service.

Novice A beginner or low-skilled player.

Offensive shot A shot designed to end a rally. Examples would include a kill shot and a pinch shot.

Order of service Determined before beginning a game; must be followed during the game.

Out Loss of service by server.

Out of court A ball that leaves the playing area.

Out of order Not following the proper order of service in doubles; results in loss of the hand.

Out serve Results in loss of service; includes non–front wall serve, touched serve, crotch serve, illegal hit, out-of-order serve, safety zone violation, 10-second violation, and fake serve.

Overhead shot Shot hit above one's head.

Pass shot A knee-high shot hit out of an opponent's reach but short of the back wall.

Pinch shot A low kill shot that hits close to the corner, either front or side wall first.

Photon A hard-hit serve.

Plum A promising set up.

Point When the receiver is not able to return a serve or makes an error in the rally; the server wins a point.

Point of contact Spot where the racquet makes contact with the ball.

Power serve Same as drive serve.

Protective eyewear Goggles or protective glasses manufactured for racquetball.

Quadriform Type of racquet head shape that favors shot placement.

Rabbit A quick player who retrieves shots all over the court.

Rally The alternating exchange of returns; continues until the end of play is caused by the ball bouncing twice or a hinder.

Ranking The ratings of competitors for tournament play.

Ready position The stance that a player takes when awaiting the next shot; the knees should be bent and the weight placed on the balls of the feet.

Receiver Player awaiting the serve.

Receiving line A line five feet behind the short line. The receiver must play the ball behind this line.

Referee Makes all decisions during the match with regard to the rules.

Reverse pinch shot A low kill shot that hits into the opposite corner of the stroke; for example, forehand shot to the left corner for a right-handed player.

Roll out A perfect kill shot that hits the front-wall floor crotch and rebounds without a bounce by rolling back into the court.

Safety hinder Occurs when a player holds up the shot in order to avoid hitting an opponent with a racquet or ball. In such cases, the point is replayed.

Safety hold up A hinder called when a player avoids action that may be hazardous to any players on the court.

Safety zone The five-foot area bounded by the back of the short line and the receiving line. This zone is observed only during the serve.

Safety zone violation Occurs when the server's partner enters the safety zone before the serve has crossed the short line. Results in loss of serve for the server.

Save Defensive shot on a ball just before it hits the floor a second time; a dig.

Screen Serve or shot that passes so close to the shooter that the receiver's view of the ball is obstructed by the hitter. During a rally it is replayed without penalty and on a serve is considered a fault.

Seniors Division Division for players at least 35 years old.

Serve Shot used to begin play.

Server The player who puts the ball in play. Only the server can score a point.

Service The right to continue serving.

Service box The 18-inch box at each end of the service area. In doubles, the server's partner must stand in this area until the serve has crossed the short line.

Service line Front line of the service area; it's 15 feet from the front wall.

Service return When the receiver returns a serve before it bounces twice on the floor.

Service zone The 5-foot by 20-foot area between the service line and the short line. The server must remain in this zone during the serve.

Set position The preparatory position between the backswing and the stroke.

Set up An easily played shot; a floater; a plum.

Short serve Fault serve that lands before passing the short line.

Short line Back line of service zone. It is at the mid-point of the court (20 feet from front wall). A legal serve must rebound past this line.

Side by side The coverage of the court used in doubles in which each player defends the 10 by 40 foot half of the court; same as half and half.

Side out Loss of service by a player or doubles team.

Side wall-front wall kill Pinch shot that hits the side wall first.

Singles Two-player game.

Skip ball Low kill shot attempt that hits the floor before it hits the front wall.

Splat An offensive shot hit from close to the side wall directly to the side wall with extreme velocity, which rebounds to the front wall and caroms at a sharp angle, making a "splat" sound.

Straight kill Same as front wall kill.

Sweet spot The center area in the stringed part of the racquet, which provides the greatest velocity to a hit.

Teardrop Type of racquet head shape that generally produces stiffer frames.

Technical A point given to a player by the referee on account of an opponent's abusive or dangerous actions.

Thong The nylon strap that is attached to the butt of the racquet and must be wrapped around the player's wrist.

Three-foot line A line in the service zone, parallel to the side wall, which limits the direction a straight drive serve may be hit.

Three-wall serve A fault serve that touches three walls before it bounces on the floor.

Throat The handle part of the racquet between the grip and the head.

Tie-breaker A game played to 11 points; used after a different player or team wins each of the first two games of a match.

Time out Each player is allowed two 30-second time outs per game.

Touch Good control of soft shots.

Touched serve A ball that hits the server when rebounding from the front wall. It is an out serve.

Tournament A formal, organized system of play to determine a champion.

Tour of the court Controlling a rally and making the opponent run all over the court.

Twinkie A game in which the losing player scores only one point.

USRA (United States Racquetball Association) The official governing body for racquetball rules, regulations, and tournament play.

Up and back See I formation.

"V" pass A cross-court passing shot that hits the side wall at the same depth as one's opponent.

Volley Hitting the ball before it bounces; a fly shot.

Wallpaper serve A serve that hugs the side wall.

Wallpaper shot A shot that hugs the side wall, making it difficult to get a good free swing at the ball.

Winner A shot that results in a point or a side out.

Wrist snap Bringing the hand through quickly as the ball is contacted, in order to add power or spin to the shot.

"Z" ball A shot that hits high on the front wall, then hits each side wall, and then hits the floor near the back wall.

"Z" lob serve Same as a "Z" serve, except it is hit high and soft.

"Z" serve A serve that hits midway up the front wall near the side wall junction, then hits the side wall, the floor, and then the other side wall near the back wall.

Index